Case Studies for Paramedics

Case Studies for Paramedics

Kevin Branch
Cambrian College

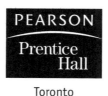

Toronto

Library and Archives Canada Cataloguing in Publication

Branch, Kevin, 1964-
　　Case studies for paramedics / Kevin Branch.

ISBN 978-0-13-207001-0

　　1. Emergency medicine--Case studies.　I. Title.

RC86.7.B73 2008　　　616.02'5　　　　C2007-905681-4

Copyright © 2009 Pearson Education Canada, a division of Pearson Canada Inc., Toronto, Ontario.

Pearson Prentice Hall. All rights reserved. This publication is protected by copyright and permission should be obtained from the publisher prior to any prohibited reproduction, storage in a retrieval system, or transmission in any form or by any means, electronic, mechanical, photocopying, recording, or likewise. For information regarding permission, write to the Permissions Department.

ISBN-13: 978-0-13-207001-0
ISBN-10: 0-13-207001-4

Vice President, Editorial Director: Gary Bennett
Acquisitions Editor: Michelle Sartor
Marketing Manager: Toivo Pajo
Developmental Editor: Pam Voves
Production Editor: Mary Ann Field
Production Coordinator: Patricia Ciardullo
Composition: Integra
Art Director: Julia Hall
Cover and Interior Design: Anthony Leung
Cover Image: Masterfile, Mike Dobel

1 2 3 4 5　　　11 10 09 08 07

Printed and bound in United States.

PEARSON Prentice Hall

All ECG readings shown in this book are from *Essentials of Paramedic Care,* Canadian Edition, by Bryan E. Bledsoe, Robert S. Porter, and Richard A. Cherry. Copyright © 2003. Reprinted by permission of Pearson Education Inc., Upper Saddle River, NJ.

Note: Knowledge and best practice in this field are constantly changing. As new research and experience broaden our knowledge, changes in practice, treatment, and drug therapy may become necessary or appropriate. Readers are advised to check the most current information provided on procedures featured or by the manufacturer of each product to be administered, to verify the recommended dose or formula, the method and duration of administration, and contraindications.

It is the responsibility of the practitioner, relying on their own experience and knowledge of the patient, to make diagnoses, to determine dosages and the best treatment for each individual patient, and to take all appropriate safety precautions. To the fullest extent of the law, neither the Publisher nor the Author assumes any liability for any injury and/or damage to persons or property arising out of or related to any use of the material contained in this book.

All characters named in these scenarios are fictional and any similarity to actual persons living or dead is coincidental.

Dedication

This text is dedicated to my family, Cathy, Brianna, and Tyler, without whom I would not be where I am today. I would like to say thanks for their patience and support in over twenty years of EMS, involving many nights away and sometimes more dedication to my career than my family.

I would also like to thank Dr. Robert Lepage, my mentor for the better part of my career, who is always motivating me to raise the bar a little higher while staying grounded, remembering who we are there for, and knowing our limitations as paramedics.

Lastly, I would like to thank my EMS colleagues and second family. I have learned firsthand that they are only a call away when needed, regardless of the situation at hand. United we still stand together, and I will always be grateful for their support.

Contents

Preface xiii

List of Abbreviations xvii

Division 1 Trauma Emergencies 1

Chapter 1 **Blunt Trauma** 1
Case 1.1 2
Case 1.2 5
Answers 7

Chapter 2 **Penetrating Trauma** 9
Case 2.1 10
Case 2.2 12
Answers 14

Chapter 3 **Hemorrhage and Shock** 17
Case 3.1 18
Case 3.2 20
Answers 23

Chapter 4 **Soft-tissue Trauma** 25
Case 4.1 26
Case 4.2 28
Answers 30

Chapter 5 **Burns** 33
Case 5.1 34
Case 5.2 36
Case 5.3 39
Answers 41

Chapter 6 **Musculoskeletal Trauma** 44
Case 6.1 45
Case 6.2 47
Answers 49

Chapter 7	**Face, Head, and Neck Trauma** 52	
	Case 7.1 53	
	Case 7.2 55	
	Answers 57	
Chapter 8	**Spinal Trauma** 60	
	Case 8.1 61	
	Case 8.2 63	
	Answers 65	
Chapter 9	**Thoracic Trauma** 68	
	Case 9.1 69	
	Case 9.2 71	
	Answers 73	
Chapter 10	**Abdominal Trauma** 75	
	Case 10.1 76	
	Case 10.2 78	
	Answers 80	

Division 2 Medical Emergencies 82

Chapter 11	**Pulmonary Emergencies** 82	
	Case 11.1 83	
	Case 11.2 85	
	Case 11.3 87	
	Case 11.4 90	
	Case 11.5 92	
	Answers 94	
Chapter 12	**Cardiology** 99	
	Case 12.1 100	
	Case 12.2 102	
	Case 12.3 104	
	Case 12.4 108	
	Answers 110	
Chapter 13	**Neurology** 114	
	Case 13.1 115	
	Case 13.2 117	

	Case 13.3	119
	Case 13.4	122
	Answers	**124**
Chapter 14	**Endocrinology**	128
	Case 14.1	129
	Case 14.2	131
	Case 14.3	133
	Answers	**135**
Chapter 15	**Allergies and Anaphylaxis**	139
	Case 15.1	140
	Case 15.2	142
	Answers	**145**
Chapter 16	**Gastroenterology**	147
	Case 16.1	148
	Case 16.2	150
	Case 16.3	152
	Case 16.4	155
	Answers	**157**
Chapter 17	**Urology and Nephrology**	161
	Case 17.1	162
	Case 17.2	164
	Answers	**166**
Chapter 18	**Toxicology and Substance Abuse**	168
	Case 18.1	169
	Case 18.2	171
	Case 18.3	174
	Case 18.4	176
	Case 18.5	178
	Case 18.6	181
	Case 18.7	183
	Case 18.8	186
	Answers	**188**
Chapter 19	**Hematology**	196
	Case 19.1	197
	Case 19.2	199
	Answers	**201**

Chapter 20	**Environmental Emergencies** 203	
	Case 20.1 204	
	Case 20.2 206	
	Case 20.3 209	
	Case 20.4 212	
	Answers 214	
Chapter 21	**Infectious Disease** 218	
	Case 21.1 219	
	Case 21.2 221	
	Answers 223	
Chapter 22	**Behavioural Disorders** 225	
	Case 22.1 226	
	Case 22.2 228	
	Case 22.3 231	
	Answers 233	
Chapter 23	**Gynecology** 237	
	Case 23.1 238	
	Case 23.2 240	
	Answers 242	
Chapter 24	**Obstetrics** 244	
	Case 24.1 245	
	Case 24.2 247	
	Case 24.3 250	
	Answers 252	

Division 3 Other Emergencies 256

Chapter 25	**Neonatology** 256	
	Case 25.1 257	
	Case 25.2 259	
	Case 25.3 261	
	Answers 264	
Chapter 26	**Pediatrics** 267	
	Case 26.1 268	
	Case 26.2 270	

	Case 26.3 272	
	Case 26.4 275	
	Case 26.5 277	
	Answers 279	
Chapter 27	**Geriatrics** 284	
	Case 27.1 285	
	Case 27.2 287	
	Answers 289	
Chapter 28	**Abuse and Assault** 292	
	Case 28.1 293	
	Case 28.2 295	
	Answers 297	
Chapter 29	**The Chronic Patient** 299	
	Case 29.1 300	
	Case 29.2 302	
	Answers 304	
Chapter 30	**Nuclear, Biological, or Chemical Assault** 306	
	Case 30.1 307	
	Answers 309	

Preface

In my years of working as a paramedic, an Advanced Care Paramedic, and then a professor, the use of treatment cases and scenarios has always come into play. Whether it was before annual certification, preceptoring students, or teaching in a classroom lab, using cases was a ritual that has continued throughout my career. This is because a case-study approach to learning reinforces the knowledge acquired as a paramedic and helps clarify the pathology learned as a student.

Although there are case study texts on the market in Canada, they do not reflect Canadian demographics or our cultural diversity. Available texts also point in the direction of American treatments and problems. As well, some texts that provide a case-study approach spend an inordinate amount of time explaining pathology and pathophysiology, or prolong a scenario over seven or eight pages.

In keeping with this scarcity of practical case study material, my own conversations with students and paramedics have made it readily apparent that they are looking for a case study text that provides current relevant scenarios, with a variety of realistic calls such as those involving street drugs.

In fact, my students and colleagues have expressed a need for cases that cover new trends of treatment and make reference to Canadian pharmacology. They have made it clear want a "meat and potatoes" approach to case studies rather than a text overloaded with pathology theory—and one that would test them through a question-and-answer format after each scenario. In writing Case Studies for Paramedics, I have ventured to provide a case study reader which meets just those needs.

I have also chosen to follow the framework of a solid Canadian paramedic textbook: Bryan Bledsoe, Robert S. Porter, Richard Cherry, & Dwayne E. Clayden's seminal Essentials of Paramedic Care, Canadian Edition. This text is valuable because of its completeness, ease of understanding, and references to Canadian Advanced Care Paramedic and Primary Care Paramedic treatments, as well as the National Occupational Competency Profile (NOCP) for paramedics. As the Essentials of Paramedic Care provides extensive coverage of anatomy, physiology, and some pathophysiology, the case study reader avoids overburdening students or paramedics by including this information.

Case Studies for Paramedics is written to complement a knowledge base of anatomy, pathophysiology, and pathology, and some cases are designed to challenge the reader to anticipate treatments. The follow-up questions relate to ECG interpretation, pharmacology, and some pathology. This text will be indispensable not onto to students, but also to working paramedics doing ongoing review, faculty members developing their own scenario ideas and evaluation tools, and ambulance service training officers studying a variety of oral scenarios.

In organizing Case Studies for Paramedics, a templated structure was chosen to provide consistency and easy reference for the reader. We of course know that paramedicine does not take a "cookbook" approach to practice, and that our assessments and treatments can go several different ways depending on unknown factors and patient involvement. However, the template structure acknowledges that, regardless of where we live in our country, we tend to assess a patient the same way. In both oral and practical scenarios there needs to be direction and consistency regarding the findings of our assessments. The template used in the text, therefore, directs the reader and provides a useful frame of reference. The treatment, whether ACP or PCP, follows the pertinent patient assessment details. A differential diagnosis concludes the case. Follow-up questions pertaining to the scenario are asked, and answers provided.

A note on regional variation and Canadian perspective: because of vast regional differences in treatments based on local policies, the NOCP was utilized for both PCP and ACP treatment. However, throughout the book references are made to every province in our country. Students and instructors alike may be able to identify familiar cities and places. Any similarity to actual addresses, emergency calls, or people (living or deceased) is, of course, purely coincidental.

I hope you will enjoy this text, whether you are using it as a student, a paramedic, or an instructor. I trust it will provide you with a useful exercise to review, or an opportunity to apply what you have learned, for this is the true intent of the text. Any comments, suggestions, reports based upon unusual situations you have encountered are always welcomed.

ACKNOWLEDGMENTS

For undertaking the task of reviewing this text and for her work and recommendations, I would like to thank Joan Desabrais, ACP. I would also like to acknowledge all the staff at Pearson Canada for their various contributions to this project.

List of Abbreviations

ABC	Airway, Breathing and Circulation	GI	Gastrointestinal
ABD	Abdomen, Abdominal	GCS	Glasgow Coma Scale
ACE	Angiotensin Converting Enzyme	GERD	Gastro-esophageal reflux disease
ACEI	Angiotensin Converting Enzyme Inhibitor	GTPAL	Gravida, Term, Premature, Abortions, Living children
ACP	Advanced Care Paramedic	H	Hydrogen
ADHD	Attention Deficit Hyperactivity Disorder	HCl	Hydrogen Chloride
A/E	Air Entry	H/N	Head and Neck
AED	Automated External Defibrillator	HCT	Hydrochlorothiazide
AGE	Arterial Gas Embolism	HHNK	Hyperglycemic Hyperosmolar Nonketotic Acidosis
ALS	Amyotrophic Lateral Sclerosis	HR	Heart Rate
ALTE	Apparent Life-Threatening Event	ICP	Intracranial Pressure
AMI	Acute Myocardial Infarction	IO	Intraosseous
APGAR	Appearance, Pulse, Grimace, Activity, Respiration	IBS	Irritable Bowel Syndrome
ATI	Acute Traumatic Ischemia	IUD	Intrauterine Device
ATV	Automated Timed Ventilator	JVD	Jugular Venous Distension
AR	Artificial Respiration	LMA	Laryngeal Mask Airway
AV	Atrioventricular	LOA	Level of Awareness
BCI	Blunt Cardiac Injury	LPM	Litres per minute (delivery of oxygen)
BP	Blood Pressure	mEq/kg	Milli-equivalents per kilogram
BPAP	Bilevel Positive Airway Pressure machine	MDI	Metered dose inhaler (used with the administration of inhaled medications, such as for asthma)
bpm	Breaths per minute (respiration) or Beats per minute (heart)	MDMA	3, 4 Methylenedioxymethamphetamine
BS	Blood Sugar	MI	Myocardial Infarction
BSA	Body Surface Area	mmol/l	Millimoles/Litre
BVM	Bag Valve mask	MVC	Motor Vehicle Collision
CC	Chief Complaint	NBCW	Nuclear, Biological and Chemical Warfare
CHF	Congestive Heart Failure	NIDDM	Non-Insulin-Dependent Diabetes Mellitus
CNO	Cannot Obtain		
COHb	Carboxyhemoglobin	NKA	No Known Allergies
CPAP	Continuous Positive Airway Pressure	NPA	Nasopharyngeal Airway
CPP	Cerebral Perfusion Pressure	NRB	Non-rebreather mask
CPR	Cardio-Pulmonary Resuscitation.	NS	Normal Saline
COPD	Chronic Obstructive Pulmonary Disease	NSAID	Non-Steroidal Anti-Inflammatory Drug
CVA	Cerebral Vascular Accident	NSR	Normal Sinus Rhythm
DCS	Decompression Sickness	NTG	Nitroglycerin
D50W	Dextrose 50% and Water	NYD	Not Yet Diagnosed
DKA	Diabetic Ketoacidosis	OPA	Oropharyngeal Airway
DNR	Do Not Resuscitate	OPP	Ontario Provincial Police
ECG	Electrocardiogram	P	Pulse
ED	Emergency Department	PAC	Premature Atrial Contraction
EMS	Emergency Medical Services	PCP	Primary Care Paramedic
ER	Emergency Room	PE	Pulmonary Embolism
ETCO2	End-Tidal-Carbon Dioxide	PEA	Pulseless Electrical Activity
ETT	Endotracheal Tube	PERL	Pupils Equal and Reactive to Light
Ext	Extremities	PICA	Posterior Inferior Cerebellar Artery

PID	Pelvic Inflammatory Disease	**SQ**	Subcutaneously
PIH	Pregnancy-Induced Hypertension	**SSRI**	Selective Serotonin Reuptake Inhibitor
PP	Pulse Pressure	**ST**	Sinus Tachycardia
PPE	Personal Protective Equipment (such as gloves, glasses, gowns, masks)	**SVT**	Supraventricular Tachycardia
		TB	Tuberculosis
PVC	Premature Ventricular Contractions	**TBSA**	Total Body Surface Area
ROM	Range of Motion	**TCA**	Tricyclic Antidepressants
RLQ	Right Lower Quadrant	**TKO**	To Keep Open
RUQ	Right Upper Quadrant	**TKVO**	To Keep Vein Open
RR	Respiratory Rate	**TdP**	Torsade de Pointes
SAED	Semi-automatic External Defibrillator	**tPA**	Tissue Plasminogen Activator
SAMPLE	Signs and Symptoms, Allergies, Medications, Past medical history, Last Meal, Events prior	**UTI**	Urinary Tract Infection
		V-Fib	Ventricular Fibrillation
		VSA	Vital Signs Absent
SCD	Sickle Cell Disease	**VT**	Ventricular Tachycardia
SIDS	Sudden Infant Death Syndrome	**Y/O**	Year Old
SNS	Sympathetic Nervous System	**YT**	Yukon Territories
SB	Shortness of Breath	**Six Ps**	Pulselessness, Pain, Pallor, Pressure, Paresthesia, and Paralysis
SPO$_2$	Saturation of Peripheral Oxygen		

Division 1 Trauma Emergencies

Chapter 1
Blunt Trauma

As with any injury, understanding the kinetics of blunt trauma is important. By obtaining a thorough incident history and understanding the injury process, paramedics can gain insight into the events preceding an accident. This information can help paramedics develop a suspicion or anticipate possible injuries and their severity. Such anticipation is paramount to an assessment, as injuries caused by blunt trauma might be hidden. It is essential to perform a rapid assessment, immobilize, and treat life threats on scene, and provide rapid transport to a trauma facility or emergency department. Any delay might jeopardize possible surgical interventions that may be required to correct the underlying conditions.

CASE 1.1

You are dispatched at 14:30hrs to a motorcycle accident on Highway 69, by the Killarney turnoff. You are familiar with this highway; its many corners and lack of passing lanes have been responsible for the loss of many lives. The weather is clear and traffic minimal. Upon arrival, you observe a 50-year-old male lying semi-prone at the base of an outcropping rock cut. Skid marks on the pavement and a point of impact on the rock cut are visible. The motorcycle is a pile of metal, some five metres away. The patient is still wearing his helmet. Bystanders on the scene tell you the accident happened at approximately 14:00hrs.

Initial Assessment Findings & Chief Complaint

LOA	Altered, but acknowledges your presence.
A	Patent, although there is blood around the patient's mouth.
B	Shallow and laboured.
C	Rapid radial pulse.
Wet Check	There is minimal blood around the patient, although the point of origin will not be known until a thorough assessment has been completed.
CC	Unable to provide this information when asked.

History

S	Abrasions, contusions, and lacerations.
A	ASA (MedicAlert).
M	digoxin, Lasix, Slow-K found in the patient's jacket pocket.
P	CNO.
L	CNO.
E	Witnesses say the patient avoided a raccoon crossing the road, progressed into a speed wobble, lost control, and hit the rock cut.

Assessment

H/N	Abrasions under right eye, 4-cm laceration to the cephalic region, abrasions on the neck.
Chest	Large contusion on sternum, asymmetrical left chest with abrasions and contusions present.
ABD	Minor abrasions.
Back	Minor abrasions.
Pelvis	Unstable.
Ext	Left leg shortened and externally rotated, with left upper arm shoulder deformity.

Vitals

BP	98/60
P	150 weak, regular
RR	26 shallow, regular
Pupils	PERL 4+ mm, slow to react
GCS	2+2+4=8
BS	5.3 mmol/l
Pulse oximetry	85%
Skin	Pale, dry

Pain Assessment

O	n/a
P	n/a
Q	n/a
R	n/a
S	n/a
T	n/a

Cardiac Monitor

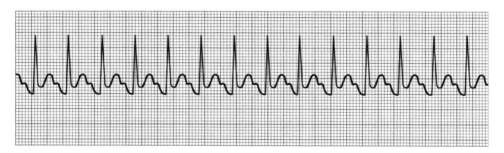

Figure 1.1

Initial Treatment Post Assessment

The patient's helmet should be removed using appropriate techniques and a c-spine immobilization should be performed utilizing a c-collar and backboard. The patient's flail chest should be stabilized with a towel and tape or large pressure dressing taped to the affected area to prevent further pleural injury. The patient must be assessed, packaged, and transported without delay. A large-bore IV should be initiated en route to the hospital. Although the patient's blood pressure is below 100/P and an IV bolus can therefore be initiated, it should be done conservatively. Oxygen should be administered via a high concentration mask. The patient's left leg should be stabilized (with a splint or secured to a backboard) and an assessment of the six Ps (pain, pulse, pallor, parathesia, paralysis, pressure) should be ongoing. The patient's mentation and vital signs should be monitored throughout transport. All lacerations and abrasions can be dressed at leisure.

En route to the trauma facility, the patient's mentation decreases and he drifts into unconsciousness. His respiratory rate slows and eventually his vital signs become absent, presenting in the following rhythm.

Cardiac Monitor

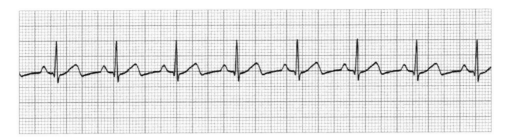

Figure 1.2

Treatment Continued

Your partner should notify medical control of the patient's deterioration as you initiate resuscitative measures. An OPA should be inserted and CPR initiated. If you are a Primary Care Paramedic (PCP) utilizing a semi-automatic AED, analysis should be completed and should result in a "No Shock Advised" prompt. Advanced Care Paramedic (ACP) treatment should include intubation and verifying ETT placement and air entry, considering the flail chest of the patient's left side. CPR should be continued and transport to a medical facility should not be delayed.

Differential Diagnosis

- Cardiac related, considering patient's history.
- Hypovolemia caused by extensive internal bleeding from impact as well as fractures in the chest and pelvis and possible abdominal injuries.
- Possible increased ICP.

Test Your Knowledge

1. Explain the meaning of the term "Golden hour" of trauma.
2. What is periorbital ecchymosis indicative of? What treatment may be contraindicated because of this finding?
3. What was the patient's rhythm upon initial assessment, and how did it change once he became VSA? What causes of the progression to VSA are in reference to this rhythm and, more specifically, to this incident?
4. Explain the pathology behind the characteristic leg-shortening and external rotation of the patient's fractured femur.
5. How does blunt trauma affect the brain?
6. What classifications are the patient's medications?

CASE 1.2

Your ambulance is dispatched at 17:15hrs to a possible quad rollover in a remote hunting camp in Northern Quebec. An old logging road leads to the site of the accident and the drive takes approximately 35 minutes. On arrival, you are met by the patient's son, who tells you that his father was coming up the hill on his quad when it rolled backward and over him. The 66-year-old father is lying supine on the hill with his feet pointing toward the top. He is still wearing his helmet. The quad is about 10 metres further down the hill.

Initial Assessment Findings & Chief Complaint

LOA	Lethargic, slightly confused.
A	Patent.
B	Regular, full volume.
C	Weak: slow, regular radial pulses.
Wet Check	Incontinent of urine.
CC	Pain in abdomen and groin.

History

S	Patient is complaining of pain in his pelvis, abdomen, and groin.
A	ASA, morphine.
M	atenolol, NTG, enalapril.
P	Hypertension, MI six years prior, angina, diet-controlled diabetes.
L	Breakfast.
E	Patient was driving his quad up a hill when it rolled back and landed on him as he fell off. No apparent loss of consciousness according to the son, but the patient bore the full weight of the quad.

Assessment

H/N	No JVD, trachea midline, pain on palpation to C-6, C-7 without obvious deformity.
Chest	Mild discomfort in lower ribs bilaterally with bruising to epigastrium.
ABD	Distended, painful on palpation of upper quadrants.
Back	Mild abrasions present on lower back, no obvious deformities.
Pelvis	Unstable on palpation.
Ext	Obvious left shoulder dislocation with good circulation and sensation; no obvious deformities in the lower or other upper extremities.

Vitals

BP	80/60
P	75 weak, regular
RR	20 shallow, regular
Pupils	PERL, 3+ mm
GCS	4+4+5=13
BS	5.2 mmol/l
Pulse oximetry	96%
Skin	Pale, diaphoretic

Pain Assessment

O	n/a
P	n/a
Q	n/a
R	n/a
S	n/a
T	n/a

Cardiac Monitor

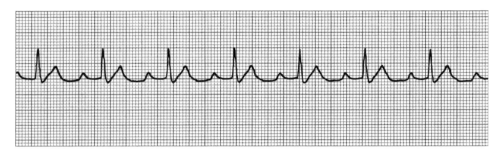

Figure 1.3

Initial Treatment Post Assessment

Treatment should include c-spine precautions and spinal immobilization after removing the patient's helmet. The patient's dislocated arm should be secured and stabilized as much as possible with a sling and swathe. Although his SPO2 is 96%, supplemental oxygen should be administered due to the potential for internal injuries and obvious fractures; for example, to the pelvis. The patient should be extricated promptly and transported without delay given the long transport time to the hospital. He may be placed in a supine position providing there is adequate respiratory effort and no obvious head injury. Air transport should be utilized if it is readily available. A large-bore IV should be initiated and a conservative bolus of 20 ml/kg infused to maintain a systolic pressure of 90–100 mm Hg. Ongoing assessment of the chest and abdomen should be done throughout transport. Because of the patient's hypotensive state and possible internal injuries, IV analgesics should not be administered.

En route to the hospital, the patient becomes more lethargic.

Differential Diagnosis

- Fractured pelvis.
- Dislocated arm.
- Possible c-spine injuries.
- Possible spleen or liver injuries.

Test Your Knowledge

1. What body systems are affected?
2. What cardiac rhythm does the patient present with?
3. The patient has low blood pressure but appears not to be compensating with an increased heart rate. Why?
4. Does the patient's age have an effect on compensatory response when he is in hypovolemic shock?
5. What classifications are the patient's medications?
6. What abdominal organs may be affected, given the presentation of a distended abdomen?

Answers

Case 1.1

1. ***Explain the meaning of the term "Golden hour" of trauma.***

   This 60-minute period begins at the impact of trauma. If surgery is required and performed within 60 minutes, the survival rate of trauma patients is significantly increased. It is important for paramedics understand that trauma patients are surgical patients, and rapid assessment, treatment, and transport are paramount for success and decreased mortality. Other modes of transport, such as air ambulance, may help in decreasing scene and transport time.

2. ***What is periorbital ecchymosis indicative of? What treatment may be contraindicated because of this finding?***

   Periorbital ecchymosis, also known as raccoon eye or black eye, is indicative of a basilar skull fracture. Because periorbital ecchymosis is caused by a hemorrhage in the base of the skull, it usually develops over time and is often not visible to paramedics during or immediately after an incident. The insertion of an NPA or nasal intubation is contraindicated in patients suspected of having a basilar skull fracture since penetration of the brain may occur by the airway adjunct. (The basal skull includes the hollow openings of sinuses, nasal cavities, auditory canals, and middle and inner ears.)

3. ***What was the patient's rhythm upon initial assessment, and how did it change once he became VSA? What causes of the progression to VSA are in reference to this rhythm and, more specifically, to this incident?***

   The patient was presenting in sinus tachycardia (ST) and progressed to Pulseless Electrical Activity (PEA), in which there are electrical complexes but no mechanical contractions of the heart. It is important to employ a structured differential diagnosis and address the probable causes of PEA, treating what is applicable to your patient. The use of the phrase 5 H's and 5 T's helps in recalling specific causes of PEA.

   5 H's
   Hypoxia
   Hypovolemia
   Hypothermia
   Hyper/hypokalemia
   Hydrogen ion (acidosis)

   5 T's
   Tablet (overdose) acidosis
   Thrombosis (coronary)
   Thrombosis (pulmonary)
   Tamponade
   Tension pneumothorax

   This patient in the scenario is likely suffering from hypoxia and hypovolemia.

4. **Explain the pathology behind the characteristic leg-shortening and external rotation of the patient's fractured femur.**

   The pathology behind the characteristic shortening and external rotation of the leg is caused by abduction of the gluteus minimus, medius, and maximus.

5. **How does blunt trauma affect the brain?**

   Blunt trauma affects the head/brain by potentially causing an increase in intracranial pressure (ICP). As pressure in the brain increases (to >20 mm Hg/cm of H_2O), cellular death can occur from cerebral herniation. Cellular death can also occur on impact, without herniation.

6. **What classifications are the patient's medications?**

digoxin (Lanoxin)	– Cardiac glycoside
Slow-K (potassium)	– Potassium supplement
Lasix (furosemide)	– Loop diuretic

Case 1.2

1. **What body systems are affected?**

Cardiovascular:	possible hypovolemia caused by the fractured pelvis and undetermined blunt trauma of the abdomen
Respiratory:	possible pulmonary contusion related to the lower rib injuries

2. **What cardiac rhythm does the patient present with?**

   The patient is presenting in a first-degree AV block.

3. **The patient has low blood pressure but appears not to be compensating with an increased heart rate. Why?**

   The patient's lack of compensation to hypotension is inappropriate. The typical sympathetic response to hypotension caused by hypovolemia is usually increased respiration and an increased heart rate. This response is not present in this patient, as his heart rate is 75 bpm. In severe hypovolemia, the end stages of shock account for the presentation of low pulse. Medics must look for other causes of mismatched vitals. The patient's skin condition and mentation is an indication of poor perfusion. The patient is on beta blockers and an Angiotensin Converting Enzyme ACE inhibitor that may be detrimental, although a sympathetic stimulation should override pharmacology.

4. **Does the patient's age have an effect on compensatory response when he is in hypovolemic shock?**

   The patient is 66 years old. Although he is not old, the compensation required in times of sympathetic stimulation is less than that of a younger patient. As we age, several effects develop specific to our body systems.

Cardiovascular:	The cardiac conduction system deteriorates and blood vessels lose the ability to constrict and dilate efficiently. In younger adults, a decrease of 1 mm Hg causes the heart rate to increase by 1 mm Hg, whereas in an elderly person it increases by 0.5 mm Hg.
Respiratory:	Gas exchange across alveolar membrane slows, causing a reduction in the ability to diffuse carbon dioxide and oxygen. The effects of hypoxia on the rate and depth of ventilation are reduced.

5. **What classifications are the patient's medications?**

atenolol (Tenormin)	– Beta blocker
NTG (Nitroglycerin)	– Nitrate, vascular smooth muscle relaxant
enalapril (Vasotec)	– ACE Inhibitor

6. **What abdominal organs may be affected, given the presentation of a distended abdomen?**

   This patient's liver and spleen are most likely affected, as he is complaining of epigastric and lower rib pain.

Chapter 2
Penetrating Trauma

The work environment of a paramedic is always changing. Incidences of penetrating traumas are on the rise, especially gunshot wounds. Knives and projectiles such as glass also cause penetrating trauma. The type of projectile or weapon used dictates whether or not sustained trauma is visible. Through scene evaluations and patient assessments, paramedics can understand the principles of energy exchange between a "weapon" and the affected body part or surrounding tissue. Penetrating trauma can also result from non-violent incidents such as sports injuries, falls, or environmental mishaps.

CASE 2.1

You are dispatched at 02:15hrs to a well-known bar on the Halifax waterfront for a possible stabbing. It is a warm night in July, and as you approach you notice a crowd has gathered outside the bar and spilled onto the city street. You see three police cars on scene. As you exit your vehicle, you are met by a police officer, who directs you to the injured party. He tells you that there is a suspect in custody in the back of a police car. The officer fills you in on the incident, stating that two teenagers, who were at the bar for several hours, began an altercation in the bar which led to a fist fight outside. Witnesses say the suspect stabbed the patient in the chest with what appeared to be a knife. The police have not found a knife on the scene.

Initial Assessment Findings & Chief Complaint

LOA	The 19-year-old patient is alert to his surroundings but appears somewhat confused about the incident. He is slurring his words.
A	Airway appears patent.
B	Shallow and laboured at 24 bpm.
C	Weak radial pulses present.
Wet Check	You observe a blood-soaked shirt with a tear in the front right chest, as well as blood on the patient's nose.
CC	Patient can't seem to catch his breath.

History

S	Shortness of breath.
A	NKA.
M	Phenytoin, Phenobarbital.
P	Epilepsy.
L	Clam strips and chips for supper.
E	Patient had been at the bar for several hours after winning money at a casino. He states he had between 12 and 15 draft beers. Another person in the bar spilled his drink, which lead to a shoving match and then a fight outside. He tells you he was fine until he felt something in his chest and couldn't catch his breath.

Assessment

H/N	Abrasions on face and epistaxis, which has now stopped.
Chest	2-cm puncture wound (bubbling) in the right anterior chest. Decreased air entry in the right lower lobe.
ABD	Soft/non-tender, unremarkable.
Back	Minor abrasions noted on upper back/shoulder.
Pelvis	Unremarkable/stable.
Ext	Abrasions on knuckles. Capillary refill delayed.

Vitals

BP	90/60
P	150
RR	24
Pupils	PERL 4+ mm
GCS	4+5+6=15
BS	n/a
Pulse oximetry	92%
Skin	Pale, diaphoretic

Pain Assessment

O	n/a
P	n/a
Q	n/a
R	n/a
S	n/a
T	n/a

Cardiac Monitor

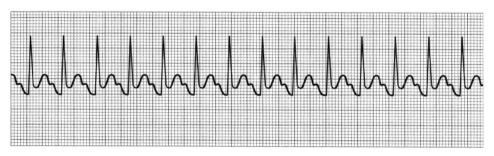

Figure 2.1

Initial Treatment Post Assessment

An initial assessment of the back and cervical spine should be completed to assess the potential for spinal immobilization. This patient had no loss of consciousness and no noted significant head trauma. Based on the incident history, the patient should be immobilized. He should receive oxygen via a high concentration mask at 12–15 lpm. The sucking chest wound should be covered with an Asherman chest seal or a three-sided occlusive dressing to prevent additional air entering the pleural cavity. The patient should be placed in a position of comfort to ease his dyspnea, with the injured side lower than the uninjured side. Transport to the emergency department should be prompt, and a large-bore IV should be initiated en route.

En route, the patient tells you that he is finding it more difficult to breathe. He appears slightly confused and says he wants to go home. He is also nauseous and fears he will vomit. You assess him further and auscultate his chest to find absent breath sounds on the right side. You observe no JVD, but the trachea appears deviated to the left. His vitals are BP 76/60, P 130 (femoral), RR 28 shallow, SP02 86%, pale and diaphoretic skin, and GCS now 3+4+6=13.

Treatment Continued

After conducting your assessment, you should remove the Asherman chest seal and examine the entry wound for any occlusion. ACP treatment should include an IV bolus of 20 ml/kg and a thoracentesis to the right chest with a Heimlich valve attached. The patient should be monitored en route to the hospital to ensure adequate ventilation. You conclude that the patient's decreased mentation may be due to hypoxia; however, because of his alcohol ingestion, blood glucometry should be performed to rule out hypoglycemia.

Blood glucometry is assessed and found to be 5.8 mmol/L.

Differential Diagnosis

- Sucking chest wound leading to a tension pneumothorax.

Test Your Knowledge

1. What is a pneumothorax?
2. What is a tension pneumothorax?
3. What are the fatal effects of a tension pneumothorax?
4. What classifications of medication is the patient taking?
5. What rhythm does the patient present with on your arrival?
6. What risk is involved when using a dressing on an open chest wound?
7. What body systems are affected in reference to the presenting patient?

CASE 2.2

You are dispatched to a summer day camp for children at Lac Saint-Jean, just outside of Dolbeau, Quebec, for an unknown problem. On arrival, you see several camp counsellors with young children varying in age from seven to 13 years old. You notice a group at the far end of a field where targets appear to be set up. As you exit your vehicle, Michel, a camp counsellor, greets you and begins to explain what happened. He is visibly upset. He tells you that during archery practice, one of the boys was accidentally shot in the leg with an arrow. The 12-year-old is in the target area and has not been moved. As you approach, you notice the patient lying supine, crying. He appears to be in a great deal of pain.

Initial Assessment Findings & Chief Complaint

LOA	Conscious/alert.
A	Patent, crying.
B	Spontaneous, appears full volume.
C	Strong radial pulses are present.
Wet Check	Approximately 10-cm radius of blood surrounding the arrow protruding through the patient's right thigh.
CC	Pain in leg.

History

S	Complaining of pain in right thigh.
A	penicillin.
M	salbutamol, Flovent.
P	Asthma.
L	Breakfast.
E	Struck by an arrow as he was walking toward the targets.

Assessment

H/N	Unremarkable.
Chest	Unremarkable, equal air entry with minimal expiratory wheezing bilaterally.
ABD	Soft/non-tender.
Back	Unremarkable.
Pelvis	Stable x3.
Ext	Upper and left lower unremarkable, arrow through right thigh with paresthesia in right leg, distal circulation, and capillary refill present bilaterally.

Vitals

BP	110/70
P	75 strong, regular
RR	22 regular, full volume
Pupils	PERL 3+ mm
GCS	4+5+6=15
BS	n/a
Pulse oximetry	99%
Skin	Pale, warm

Pain Assessment

O	n/a
P	n/a
Q	n/a
R	n/a
S	n/a
T	n/a

Cardiac Monitor

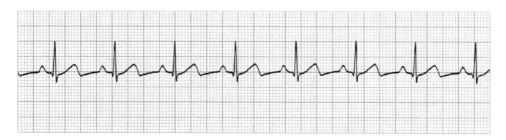

Figure 2.2

Initial Treatment Post Assessment

C-spine assessment should be performed to rule out any other trauma. Once c-spine has been ruled out, the penetrating arrow needs to be secured in place with pressure dressings on the entrance and exit openings. Because of the location of the wound, the age of the child, and the pain he is in, the arrow needs to be adequately secured to prevent further injury. The patient should be transported in a semi-prone position. An intravenous should be initiated and run at TKO.

En route to the medical facility, the patient complains of more pain in the affected extremity as well as numbness. Pedal pulses are present bilaterally. Capillary refill is normal in all extremities. Expiratory wheezing increases and the patient becomes more apprehensive.

Treatment Continued

Reassessment of the patient's leg should continue en route. Administration of salbutamol 900 μg MDI or 5.0 mg nebulized can be administered to relieve wheezing and help decrease respiratory distress caused by trauma and anxiety. Analgesia should be considered for isolated extremity injuries in the absence of hypotension.

Differential Diagnosis

- Penetrating trauma in right thigh.
- Asthma.

Test Your Knowledge

1. How should the arrow be stabilized?
2. How should the patient be positioned on a stretcher for transport?
3. What complications can occur from having an arrow in the thigh?
4. What further assessments should be carried out en route to the hospital?
5. What classifications of medications is the patient on?
6. Why should the arrow not be removed?
7. What might be causing the paresthesia in the patient's affected leg?
8. What ECG does the patient present with?

Answers

Case 2.1

1. *What is a pneumothorax?*

    A pneumothorax occurs when air enters the pleural cavity. It can be spontaneous or the result of blunt force trauma to the chest. Air enters the pleural cavity from the airways; higher pressure in the alveolar tissue allows air to move into the pleural cavity, which causes the lung to collapse.

2. *What is a tension pneumothorax?*

    A tension pneumothorax occurs when air leaks into the pleural cavity during inspiration and cannot leave. Pressure eventually builds and causes the mediastinum to shift to the unaffected side. Minimal air enters the affected lung through the airway as a result of its collapse, which eventually leads to hypoxia, decreased ventilation, and perfusion.

3. *What are the fatal effects of a tension pneumothorax?*

   The fatal effects of a tension pneumothorax are hypoxemia and decreased perfusion. Pressure caused by increased air or blood in the pleural cavity can affect heart function and cause a patient to become hypotensive. The patient may also present with jugular vein distension (JVD) in the absence of hypovolemia.

4. *What classifications of medication is the patient taking?*

   phenytoin (Dilantin)   – Anti-convulsant
   phenobarbital (phenobarb) – Barbiturate

5. *What rhythm does the patient present with on your arrival?*

   The patient is presenting in sinus tachycardia.

6. *What risk is there when using a dressing on an open chest wound?*

   There is a real risk of occluding a sucking chest wound with a dressing or chest seal, since this kind of dressing has the potential to cause a tension pneumothorax. (A tension pneumothorax occurs when air in the pleural space cannot exit and pressure increases within the cavity.) If, post treatment, assessment dictates that a chest injury is progressing to a tension pneumothorax, the occlusive dressing should be removed. An audible escape of air may then be heard. Once removed, if signs and symptoms do not subside, the wound should be assessed for possible closure due to fluid or blood. If sealed, and if local protocols dictate, the wound should be gently spread open, allowing the build-up of air to escape.

7. *What body systems are affected in reference to the presenting patient?*

   Respiratory and cardiovascular (circulatory) systems are affected in this patient.

Case 2.2

1. *How should the arrow be stabilized?*

   The arrow should be stabilized using large pressure dressings to surround the arrow and minimize movement. Both sides of the thigh should be packed and stabilized, secured with tape or another adhesive.

2. *How should the patient be positioned on a stretcher for transport?*

   The patient should be positioned semi-prone with the affected leg supported by the uninjured leg. This positioning should provide stabilization and allow for additional assessment of the patient en route to the hospital. Care should be taken to ensure safe loading and unloading of the patient so that the arrow does not catch on blankets and door jambs.

3. *What complications can occur from having an arrow in the thigh?*

   Several complications can occur from penetrating injuries involving the thigh. As it is large area of the axial skeleton, internal bleeding is possible. Neural damage can occur, affecting mobility and/or causing paresthesia, particularly involving the posterior femoral cutaneous nerve, sciatic nerve, or saphenous nerve. Later complications may also include infection.

4. *What further assessments should be carried out en route to the hospital?*

   The affected extremity should be continually assessed for the six Ps.

Pain:	reassessment of pain in the affected extremity
Pallor:	reassessment of the colour of the extremity including capillary refill
Paresthesia:	reassessment for continued numbness or tingling in the extremity
Paralysis:	reassessment of the patient's ability to move the leg distal to the penetration
Pressure:	reassessment of increased tension within the extremity
Pulses:	reassessment of dorsalis pedis or posterial tibialis

5. *What classifications of medications is the patient on?*

   salbutamol (Ventolin) — Bronchodilator, beta adrenergic
   Flovent (fluticasone propionate) — Corticosteroid

6. *Why should the arrow not be removed?*

   Because of the potential for increased nerve and vascular damage, the arrow should not be removed until an X-ray can be taken. Removal of the arrow might further damage vascular areas of the leg and cause increased bleeding, which may currently be tamponaded by the arrow.

7. *What might be causing the paresthesia in the patient's affected leg?*

   Paresthesis may be caused by severing or partial severing of the saphenous, posterior femoral cutaneous, or sciatic nerve. Also, due to blood loss from the leg, compartment syndrome may develop, increasing pressure on the affected nerves despite their not having sustained any specific trauma.

8. *What ECG does the patient present with?*

   The patient presents in a normal sinus rhythm.

Chapter 3
Hemorrhage and Shock

While the loss of blood through hemorrhage is a life threat, the progression to the lack of oxygenation and perfusion, known as shock, is a serious condition. The signs and symptoms of internal bleeding can be subtle and progress rapidly over time. A careful assessment of the mechanism of injury and a thorough assessment of the patient can help paramedics recognize the potential for life-threatening injuries. For patients suffering from hemorrhage or shock, rapid assessment and prompt transport to a medical facility are paramount. Treatment on scene, and particularly en route, may be aggressive, including oxygenation and fluid resuscitation. In a patient presenting in hypovolemic shock, the goal of treatment is the maintenance of vital signs. A patient's chances for survival will be greatly improved with the progression of care en route to the hospital.

CASE 3.1

You are dispatched to a local bar at 01:20hrs on 1400 Rue Sainte-Catherine Ouest, Montreal. The police are on scene, and through dispatch you are advised that a young male, twenty-seven years old, has put his fist through a window. On arrival, the patient is leaning against a police cruiser. His right hand is wrapped in a towel saturated with blood. As you survey the scene, you see that the window he has punched is a typical glass door piped with metal strands. The police inform you that the patient's name is Paolo, and that he has had a few drinks. Apparently, Paolo had been in a dispute with a friend inside the bar, was asked to leave, and punched the glass door on the way out. The bouncer came outside, attempted to stop the bleeding, and called 911. Paolo is pale and compliant to treatment.

Initial Assessment Findings & Chief Complaint

LOA	Conscious but confused.
A	Patent.
B	Shallow.
C	Weak radial pulses.
Wet Check	Gross bleed from the right forearm.
CC	Laceration.

History

S	Patient sustained laceration on the right wrist.
A	None.
M	Ativan.
P	Anxiety.
L	Supper.
E	The patient was upset with a friend in the bar, and as he was leaving, punched a metal-reinforced window. He began bleeding, and the bouncer wrapped his arm in a towel and called 911.

Assessment

H/N	Unremarkable.
Chest	Unremarkable, equal air entry bilaterally.
ABD	Soft/non-tender.
Back	Unremarkable.
Pelvis	Stable.
Ext	Lower extremities unremarkable; right forearm sustained an approximately 7-cm by 3-cm avulsion on the medial aspect with squirting bright red blood. The patient's capillary refill is delayed.

Vitals

BP	80/60
P	150, regular
RR	24
Pupils	PERL 4+ mm, slow
GCS	4+4+6=14
BS	4.8 mmol/l
Pulse oximetry	100%
Skin	Pale, diaphoretic

Pain Assessment

O	20 minutes
P	Broken window
Q	Sore
R	None
S	7/10
T	20 minutes

Cardiac Monitor

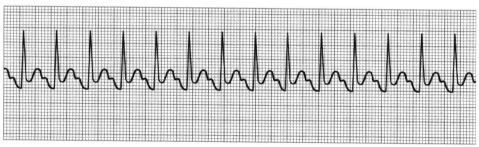

Figure 3.1

Initial Treatment Post Assessment

An initial assessment and documented mechanism of injury should be completed to rule out the need for c-spine precautions. A baseline set of vitals should be obtained, including SPO2 and a blood glucometry. Oxygen should be administered via a high concentration mask. The towel should be removed from the patient's arm after large and small pressure dressings have been unwrapped and made available for use. Due to the arterial bleed from the forearm, a large pressure dressing should be tightly secured over the injury. Transport to the hospital should be prompt and scene time kept to a minimum. En route, an intravenous should be established and a 20 ml/kg IV bolus initiated. The patient should be positioned supine or in a position of comfort.

En route, you observe blood seeping through the pressure dressing on the arm. The patient is still pale, and his vitals remain the same as on scene.

Treatment Continued

An additional pressure dressing should be placed on the existing dressing. The original dressing should not be removed. The patient's mentation and vital signs should be monitored during transport. The intravenous bolus should continue after the original 600 ml have infused.

Differential Diagnosis

- Arterial bleed.
- Hypovolemia (hemorrhagic shock).

Test Your Knowledge

1. Based on the patient's presentation, how much blood do you anticipate he lost prior to your arrival?
2. As the body attempts to compensate for blood loss, what stages of shock does it enter and progress through?
3. How many litres of blood would a typical 70-kg patient have?
4. What are the three steps of the clotting process for a patient with a local hemorrhage?
5. What ECG does the patient present with?
6. What is the classification of the patient's medication?
7. Why is a tourniquet a last resort in an attempt to stop a life-threatening hemorrhage?

CASE 3.2

On a quiet Sunday night in June, and you are dispatched at 20:00hrs to a motor vehicle accident on Beaver Brook Road, Miramichi. As you pull up to the scene, you realize your predictions were right: a car has struck a moose out for an evening stroll. You observe that the car has gone off the road, and there is a lone occupant in the driver's seat. There is extensive damage to the front end and roof of the car but the area appears secure and safe. Judging from the damage, it appears the moose was hit and knocked up and over the car. You see the moose lying motionless on the road and consider it fortunate that it was not full-grown: a moose can weigh up to 450 kg and stand two metres tall. The driver is alert, pale, and diaphoretic. She tells you that both her legs are painful to move. She also tells you that she is pregnant and due in one month.

Initial Assessment Findings & Chief Complaint

LOA	Slightly confused.
A	Patent.
B	Regular and full volume.
C	Weak radial pulses present.
Wet Check	Mild bleeding from forehead.
CC	Leg trauma.

History

S	Patient is complaining of leg pain.
A	None.
M	Materna, folic acid.
P	Healthy and 36 weeks pregnant.
L	Supper at 18:00hrs.
E	Patient was driving home, struck a moose in the middle of the road, and drove off the road.

Assessment

H/N	No JVD, trachea midline, complaining of mild lateral neck pain.
Chest	Mild abrasion on epigastric area from steering wheel.
ABD	Soft/non-tender.
Back	Unremarkable.
Pelvis	Stable.
Ext	Bilateral femur fractures and right ankle deformity. Capillary refill is delayed.

Vitals

BP	88/68
P	150
RR	26 full volume
Pupils	PERL 3+ mm
GCS	4+5+6=15
BS	6.8 mmol/l
Pulse oximetry	96%
Skin	Pale and diaphoretic

Pain Assessment

O	n/a
P	n/a
Q	n/a
R	n/a
S	n/a
T	n/a

Cardiac Monitor

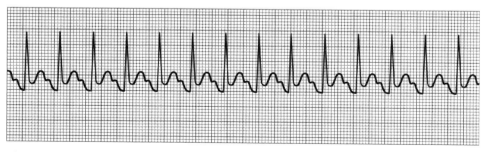

Figure 3.2

Initial Treatment Post Assessment

The patient should be assessed while c-spine support is maintained. Oxygen should be administered via a high concentration mask. The patient should have a c-collar applied, and rapid extrication techniques should be used to transfer her from the vehicle onto a fracture board. She should be secured to the board and transported to the waiting ambulance. Once on the stretcher, the patient's legs should be assessed distally for circulation and sensation and secured to prevent further injury. The use of a traction splint is questionable because of the hemodynamical instability of the patient and her pregnancy. A complete set of vitals should be obtained, including SPO2, ECG interpretation, and blood glucometry. The patient should then be placed in a left lateral recumbent position, with padding under one side of the fracture board. An intravenous should be initiated en route to the hospital and a 20 ml/kg bolus infused. Transportation should be prompt and scene time minimized.

En route, the patient remains pale and diaphoretic and maintains a blood pressure of 94/60 with 500 ml of IV fluid infused.

Treatment Continued

Constant re-evaluation of the patient and fetus should occur, and the IV bolus should be continued. ACP treatment for this trauma patient is the same.

Differential Diagnosis

- Bilateral femur fracture.
- Hypovolemic shock.
- Possible fetal hypoxemia.

Test Your Knowledge

1. What might paramedics anticipate, based on the mechanism of injury?
2. Given the patient's presentation and injuries, approximately how much blood might she have lost?
3. Although this patient is presenting with symptoms of shock, why might the signs be delayed in a pregnant patient?
4. Why might a fetus be compromised in a hypovolemic situation such as this?
5. What are the classifications of the patient's medications?
6. What ECG does the patient present with?
7. Based on the patient's vital signs and presentation, what class of shock is she presenting in?

Answers
Case 3.1

1. ***Based on the patient's presentation, how much blood do you anticipate he lost prior to your arrival?***

    The patient is somewhat confused, pale, diaphoretic with a BP of 80/60, and has a compensatory heart rate of 150. He has lost approximately 25–35% of his blood and is in stage 3 (class 3) decompensated shock.

2. ***As the body attempts to compensate for blood loss, what stages of shock does it enter and progress through?***

    The body attempts to compensate for blood loss with four stages of shock.

Compensated shock (Stage 1 and 2):	Initial stage
	Pulse rate increases
	Pulse strength decreases
	Skin becomes cool and clammy
	Increased anxiety and restlessness
	Thirst and weakness become apparent
Decompensated shock (Stage 3):	Begins when the body can no longer compensate
	Pulse becomes unpalpable
	Blood pressure drops
	Patient becomes unconscious
	Respirations slow or cease
Irreversible shock (Stage 4):	Lack of circulation has a profound effect on the body
	Cells die
	Tissues dysfunction
	Organs dysfunction
	Patient dies

3. ***How many litres of blood would a typical 70-kg patient have?***

    70 kg × 70 ml/kg = 4900 ml
    The patient in question would have approximately five litres of blood.

4. ***What are the three steps of the clotting process for a patient with a local hemorrhage?***

    The three stages of the clotting process are the vascular phase, platelet phase, and coagulation.

Vascular phase:	As a blood vessel is torn, the smooth muscle contracts, making the lumen smaller.
Platelet phase:	As platelets adhere to the vessel walls, they "aggregate" or collect other platelets.
Coagulation:	Enzymes are released into the blood, triggering a series of chain reactions, which result in fibrin production. Other processes continue until the wound is drawn together.

5. ***What ECG does the patient present with?***

    The patient is presenting in a sinus tachycardia.

6. ***What is the classification of the patient's medication?***

    Ativan (lorazepam) — Benzodiazepine

7. ***Why is a tourniquet a last resort in an attempt to stop a life-threatening hemorrhage?***

    A tourniquet is a last resort because if a tourniquet is applied, blood becomes stagnant and lactic acid, potassium, and other anaerobic metabolites accumulate. When or if the tourniquet is released, these toxins enter central circulation and may have devastating results. In addition, the tourniquet occludes all blood flow to distal circulation, therefore making the area ischemic.

Case 3.2

1. *What might paramedics anticipate, based on the mechanism of injury?*

   Paramedics should anticipate the presence of shock rather than waiting for overt signs. This patient is presenting with pallor and diaphoresis, and is already in a substantial degree of shock.

2. *Given the patient's presentation and injuries, approximately how much blood might she have lost?*

   The patient is presenting with bilateral femur fractures and a possible fracture to her ankle. Therefore, she may have lost approximately 1500–2000 ml of blood because of reduced pressure in the thigh.

3. *Although this patient is presenting with symptoms of shock, why might the signs be delayed in a pregnant patient?*

   Signs and symptoms of shock may be delayed in a pregnant patient because of the increased blood volume during pregnancy. Approximately 30–35% blood loss can occur before signs and symptoms of shock appear.

4. *Why might a fetus be compromised in a hypovolemic situation such as this?*

   With severe blood loss, significant vasoconstriction can occur in response to catecholamine release. Also, 10–20% of normal uterine blood flow is shunted away from the uterus to aid in compensation of maternal shock.

5. *What are the classifications of the patient's medications?*

   Materna (Materna) – Vitamin preparation for pregnancy
   folic acid (Folic Acid) – Vitamin B complex

6. *What ECG does the patient present with?*

   The patient is presenting in a sinus tachycardia.

7. *Based on the patient's vital signs and presentation, what class of shock is she presenting in?*

   With a 30–35% blood loss, the patient is presenting in class 3 bordering on class 4 shock.

Chapter 4
Soft-tissue Trauma

In the presentation of soft-tissue injury, damage occurs to the skin—the outer layer of protection of the body. When skin continuity is breached, there is an increased potential of injury to internal organs, because the breach may hamper the body's ability to contain the organs and maintain circulating blood volume. Recognition of soft-tissue injuries and the potential for internal injury is therefore essential. However, discoloration may not be obvious at the initial time of assessment but may occur later. By determining the mechanism of injury, potential injuries may be anticipated even though they are not apparent. With soft-tissue damage, stabilizing and immobilizing the injured site will prevent further injury and aid the patient's recovery.

CASE 4.1

At 13:45hrs, you are dispatched to a possible explosion involving a road crew member on the Stewart-Cassiar Highway in British Columbia. On arrival, you see that the highway surrounding the road construction site is closed. You are directed to the far side of the site, where you are met by the site foreman and patient. The patient, 58-year-old Edward, was apparently planting charges for rock blasting when a blasting cap went off in his hand. There was no loss of consciousness, and the injuries are isolated to his hands and forearms. He is sitting on the side of the road with his hands wrapped in towels.

Initial Assessment Findings & Chief Complaint

LOA	Conscious and alert.
A	Patent.
B	Regular and full volume.
C	Radial pulses present.
Wet Check	Towel on the left hand is saturated with blood.
CC	Blast injury on hands.

History

S	Complains of pain in both hands.
A	None.
M	ASA, cyclobenzaprine, 222 (ASA, caffeine, and codeine), Tylenol.
P	Heart problems, ongoing back pain, pacemaker.
L	Lunch.
E	The patient was planting blasting caps in the rocks for road work when a blasting cap went off in his hand. He was dropped back on his buttocks on the rock from the force of the blast, but there was no loss of consciousness.

Assessment

H/N	No JVD, trachea midline, no obvious trauma noted.
Chest	Unremarkable, equal air entry bilaterally.
ABD	Soft/non-tender.
Back	Unremarkable.
Pelvis	Stable.
Ext	Lower extremities unremarkable. Left hand has multiple abrasions, avulsions with an amputation of the thumb and index finger with protruding bone and minimal bleeding. The patient wears a wedding ring on his ring finger. His right hand is red and swollen with minor abrasions present.

Vitals

BP	130/88
P	75, regular
RR	20
Pupils	PERL 3+ mm
GCS	4+5+6=15
BS	n/a
Pulse oximetry	98%
Skin	Warm, diaphoretic

Pain Assessment

O	Sudden
P	Blasting cap
Q	Sharp, numb
R	None
S	10/10
T	30 minutes

Cardiac Monitor

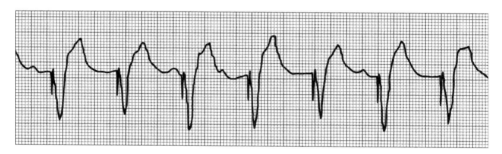

Figure 4.1

Initial Treatment Post Assessment

Initial assessment should involve ruling out c-spine injury and ensuring airway patency. Vitals, including SPO2, should be obtained by your partner while you attend to the patient's wounds. Because of the injury to the patient's left hand, you should attempt to remove his ring. A dressing such as a 4 × 4 with kling should be wrapped around the affected remnants of the injured digits and around the left hand. Assess, clean, and dress the right hand. Capillary refill should be assessed in both hands for distal circulation, and both hands should be elevated. Oxygen should be administered via a low concentration device and ECG monitoring should ensue. An intravenous should be initiated and run at TKVO en route to the hospital. An ACP should administer narcotic analgesics for pain management if needed.

En route, the patient complains of increased pain and weakness in his right hand as well as decreased touch sensation in his fingers. Both hands are swollen, but the right is extremely swollen and appears to be growing in front of your eyes.

Treatment Continued

Assessment of the patient's hands should continue with emphasis on circulation and sensation. A cold compress and elevation may benefit the edema of the right hand. Rapid transport is key for this patient. Narcotic analgesics should continue to be administered by an ACP.

Differential Diagnosis

- Amputation.
- Compartment syndrome in right hand.

Test Your Knowledge

1. What is compartment syndrome?
2. What is the usual cause of compartment syndrome?
3. The patient's right hand is presenting with minimal visible trauma, yet has more edema than the left. Why?
4. What are the signs and symptoms of compartment syndrome?
5. What parts of the body are usually affected by compartment syndrome?
6. What ECG does the patient present with?
7. What are the classifications of the patient's medications?

CASE 4.2

At 13:45hrs, you are dispatched to an old hunting camp off a popular climbing hill at Minister's Face, New Brunswick, for a trapped patient. The local volunteer fire department is also responding to the call. En route, dispatch advises you that climbers found an approximately 45-year-old man screaming for help at the camp. The patient is trapped under a camp wall he was working on. The climbers are trying to dig him out, but the wall sections are too heavy for them. As you arrive with the fire truck behind you, you observe the scene as described. The man, named Jocelyn, tells you that once the wall came down he was sure he would die. It has covered him from the waist down. He is conscious but mildly disoriented as to time. He tells you that his legs are pinned and he can't get them out. Jocelyn says his legs were extremely sore shortly after the wall toppled but that now he is not sure how his legs feel as he has lost all sensation.

Initial Assessment Findings & Chief Complaint

LOA	Conscious with mild confusion.
A	Patent.
B	Normal.
C	Strong radial pulse.
Wet Check	Unremarkable in the areas that can be seen.
CC	Crush injury to legs.

History

S	Complains of numbness in lower legs.
A	ASA.
M	Synthroid, fluoxetine, amitriptyline, Tylenol 3.
P	Thyroid disorders, migraines, mild depression.
L	Lunch.
E	The patient was reinforcing a wall in an old hunting camp when it crashed down on him. He attempted to run, but was knocked down and trapped as the wall collapsed. Afterward, he attempted to wiggle his way out, but was in too much pain to make any progress.

Assessment

H/N	Unremarkable, no JVD, trachea midline.
Chest	Unremarkable, with equal air entry bilaterally.
ABD	Soft/non-tender.
Back	Unremarkable (what can be assessed).
Pelvis	Appears stable.
Ext	Upper extremities unremarkable. Lower extremities trapped under wall and cannot be assessed.

Vitals

BP	126/86
P	60, regular
RR	14
Pupils	PERL 3+ mm
GCS	4+4+6=15
BS	5.1 mmol/l
Pulse oximetry	98%
Skin	Warm and dry

Pain Assessment

O	1 hour
P	Crushing
Q	Numbness
R	None
S	Cannot assign severity
T	1 hour

Cardiac Monitor

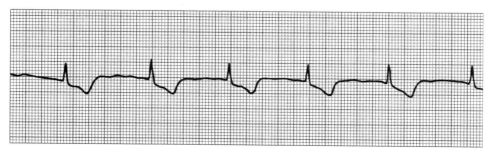

Figure 4.2

Initial Treatment Post Assessment

Initial treatment of this incident should centre on scene safety and securing the wall to prevent injury to paramedics, firefighters, or bystanders, or further injury to the patient. Once secured, c-spine immobilization should be maintained until the patient is assessed. Oxygen should be administered via a high concentration mask. A thorough assessment should be performed on accessible areas. Vital signs should be obtained, including SPO2, blood glucometry, and ECG interpretation. A cervical collar should be applied and an intravenous secured and run at TKVO until just prior to the removal of the trapped patient. As an ACP, medical direction should be consulted and the administration of Sodium Bicarbonate may be beneficial to the patient.

Approximately 25 minutes after arriving on scene, the wall is lifted and secure enough to allow Jocelyn to be removed.

Treatment Continued

The patient should be slid onto a fracture board and secured, and rapid transport should be initiated. Intravenous boluses should continue en route to the hospital as long as the lung fields are clear of pulmonary edema.

Differential Diagnosis

- Crush injury to the legs.

Test Your Knowledge

1. Upon your arrival on scene, what do you notice that is significant about the patient's position?
2. What are the usual complaints of a trapped patient?
3. What prevents the patient from experiencing the effects of crush injury?
4. If fluid bolusing is not available, what treatment may be considered?
5. What ECG does the patient present with?
6. What term for crush injuries focuses attention on the underlying problem, and is therefore preferred?
7. What classifications are the patient's medications?

Answers

Case 4.1

1. *What is compartment syndrome?*

    Compartment syndrome occurs when tissue pressures in a confined space increase to the point of compromising the perfusion of the affected area.

2. **What is the usual cause of compartment syndrome?**

   Compartment syndrome is usually caused by increased arterial and venous pressures at the capillary level. As pressure within a compartment increases, tissue perfusion is compromised by loss of vasomotor tone or collapse of veins. Elevated compartment pressure can be caused by a hematoma forming in a closed compartment or by accumulating edema.

3. **The patient's right hand is presenting with minimal visible trauma, yet has more edema than the left. Why?**

   The right hand sustained injury caused by the pressure wave created by the blasting cap explosion in the left hand. Although it had only minor abrasions, the right hand received more tissue damage, resulting in edema formation. While the left hand sustained injuries from the pressure wave, two fingers were also amputated (removed), thus creating an external area for fluid to shift without causing compartmentalizing.

4. **What are the signs and symptoms of compartment syndrome?**

   Signs and symptoms of compartment syndrome include the following:
   Mechanism of injury suggestive of compartment syndrome
   Increased pain
   Decreased touch sensation
   Increased weakness of the affected area
   Increased pallor and swelling
   Decreased pulses and capillary refill

5. **What parts of the body are usually affected by compartment syndrome?**

   The parts of the body usually affected by compartment syndrome include all extremities, but most often the lower arm, hand, lower leg, and foot.

6. **What ECG does the patient present with?**

   The patient is presenting with a paced rhythm.

7. **What are the classifications of the patient's medications?**

ASA (acetylsalicylic acid)	– NSAID
Flexeril (cyclobenzaprine)	– Skeletal muscle relaxant
222 (ASA with codeine)	– Narcotic analgesic
Tylenol (acetaminophen)	– Analgesic

Case 4.2

1. **Upon your arrival on scene, what do you notice that is significant about the patient's position?**

   The patient is trapped under a hunting camp wall constructed of brick, metal, and wood. The wall, which is extremely heavy, has fallen across the patient's lower extremities. The patient is supine and his upper body appears unremarkable.

2. **What are the usual complaints of a trapped patient?**

   The usual complaints of entrapment or crushing syndromes include the following:
   Pain
   Lack of motor function
   Tingling
   Loss of sensation in the affected limb
   Sensory loss of the limb
   Paralysis

3. **What prevents the patient from experiencing the effects of crush injury?**

   As long as the body parts are trapped, the patient will not experience the true effects of crush syndrome, such as the release of toxic byproducts into circulation.

4. *If fluid bolusing is not available, what treatment may be considered?*

    If fluid bolusing is not available, consider applying a tourniquet before the trapped pressure is released. This will hold the toxins and prevent reperfusion injury.

5. *What ECG does the patient present with?*

    The patient is presenting with a junctional escape rhythm.

6. *What term for crush injuries focuses attention on the underlying problem, and is therefore preferred?*

    The term Acute Traumatic Ischemia (ATI) focuses attention on the underlying problem of crush injuries and is therefore preferred.

7. *What classifications are the patient's medications?*

Synthroid (levothyroxine)	– Thyroid agent
Prozac (fluoxetine)	– Antidepressant
Elavil (amitriptyline)	– Antidepressant
Tylenol 3 (acetaminophen with codeine 30 mg)	– Analgesic

Chapter 5
Burns

The protective covering of the body—the skin—is compromised by burns. This compromise may in turn weaken the body's ability to be a contained entity, causing the loss of valuable fluids. As well, compromise of the skin provides an opportunity for foreign agents to enter. Intervention to prevent undue exposure is important in the assessment and treatment of burn patients. Assessments should be prompt, and an intervention of treatment to stop the burning process should be initiated. Determination of a burn's depth is important in recommending treatment. Careful attention should be paid to the location of the burn, particularly in the areas of the chest, neck, and face. Compromise to breathing and airways should be anticipated with these locations. Finally, fluid resuscitation is important for severe burns.

CASE 5.1

You are dispatched priority 4 to a house fire at 34 8th Street, Luseland, Saskatchewan. It is a dark July night as you glance at the clock, which shows 02:50hrs. Upon arrival, you observe two firefighters attending to a female child on the front lawn of a residence that is fully engulfed in flames. There are many firefighters on scene, and the air is thick with black smoke. The firefighters advise you that the 10-year-old was hiding in a closet when they found her, and that the fire began in the room adjacent to hers. They carried her out and have begun to remove some of her burned clothing.

Initial Assessment Findings & Chief Complaint

LOA	Conscious, alert, frightened.
A	Patent, with soot around the mouth and nose.
B	Shallow and laboured.
C	Strong radial pulses present.
Wet Check	No bodily fluids but extensive burns to chest, abdomen, and arms.
CC	Dyspnea and pain to affected areas.

History

S	The patient is complaining of difficulty breathing and extreme pain in the chest and other burned areas.
A	Sulpha drugs, cigarette smoke.
M	Theophylline, carbamazapine.
P	Asthma, epilepsy.
L	Supper last night.
E	The patient was sleeping and awoke coughing because of the smoke in the room. She tried to leave the bedroom, sustaining burns in the process. She then hid in the closet to escape the flames.

Assessment

H/N	Soot noted around the mouth and nose. Second-degree burns on anterior neck.
Chest	Third-degree burns on upper chest, second-degree burns on lower chest. Upon auscultation, there is audible wheezing bilaterally to the apexes and crackles to the bilateral bases.
ABD	First-degree burns on the entire abdomen.
Back	Unremarkable.
Pelvis	Stable x3.
Ext	First-degree burns on both upper arms (anterior only). Capillary refill delayed. Skin cool with the exception of affected areas.

Vitals

BP	100/70
P	150, regular
RR	10, shallow
Pupils	PERL 3 mm
GCS	4+5+6=15
BS	n/a
Pulse oximetry	88%
Skin	Cool to touch

Pain Assessment

O	n/a
P	n/a
Q	n/a
R	n/a
S	n/a
T	n/a

Cardiac Monitor

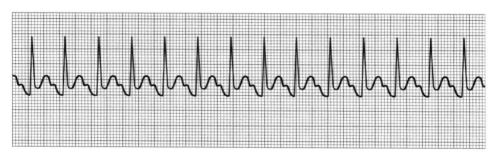

Figure 5.1

Initial Treatment Post Assessment

The patient's burned and smouldering clothing should be removed to stop the burning process and allow appropriate assessment. Oxygen saturation (although not relevant in possible CO poisoning), a CO monitor, and oxygen should be administered promptly via a non-rebreather mask NRB at 12–15 lpm. The patient should then be placed in a position of comfort in the ambulance. First-degree burns on the patient's chest, arms, and abdomen should be treated with damp dressings. The remainder of the burns, those third-degree in severity, should be dressed with dry dressings. If transport time is relatively short, damp dressings may also be used on the third-degree burns. Salbutamol 900 μg MDI or 5.0 mg nebulized salbutamol should be administered to aid the patient's dyspnea and expiratory wheezing. An IV should be initiated and run at TKVO. An IV bolus may exacerbate the patient's pulmonary edema. Analgesics should be avoided or used cautiously as the patient's blood pressure is 100/70.

En route to the hospital, the patient experiences a tonic-clonic seizure and remains unconscious with shallow respirations of 4 bpm. There is no significant change in the patient's ECG.

Treatment Continued

Post-seizure suctioning should ensure airway patency, and an airway adjunct such as an OPA or laryngeal mask should be utilized if the patient remains unconscious. Ventilations should be assisted with a bag-valve-mask, ensuring appropriate tidal volume as compliance is impaired. An ACP should consider intubation (ETT no. 6.5, 19.5 cm at the teeth). If compliance does not improve and there is still evidence of bronchoconstriction, additional dosages of salbutamol should be considered. Blood glucometry should be assessed post-seizure (4.1 mmol/l).

Differential Diagnosis

- Inhalation injuries causing respiratory distress.
- First-, second- and third-degree burns.
- Hypoxia.

Test Your Knowledge

1. Using the "Rule of Nines," what is the approximate total burned body surface area on this patient?
2. Describe the pathology of shock in burn patients.
3. Would this patient's burns be considered major, moderate, or minor?
4. Why was compliance poor while ventilating this child?
5. Why would you not want to cool a second-degree burn that is more extensive than 10–15%?
6. On arrival at the hospital, fluid resuscitation should be initiated. Using the Parkland Burn Formula, how much fluid should be infused over a 24-hour period?
7. What classifications of medications is the patient on?
8. What ECG does the patient present with?

CASE 5.2

You are dispatched at 22:00hrs to Tobin Lake, just north of Nipawin, Saskatchewan, for a patient with possible burns. On arrival you are greeted by a neighbour, who directs you to the patient. He tells you that Kris was lighting a bonfire using gasoline and the bonfire flamed up as he ignited it. The neighbour tells you that the flames were approximately two metres high and hit Kris in the face and chest. The neighbour also tells you that a group of friends had been drinking and no one was sober enough to drive to the hospital so they called 911. Kris is pacing back and forth some distance from the fire, in obvious pain.

Initial Assessment Findings & Chief Complaint

LOA	Kris is alert as to time and place but appears confused regarding the actual incident and how he was burned. He has an unsteady gait and staggers as you try to talk with him.
A	Patent with obvious burns surrounding the mouth and face. There is a strong smell of what appears to be alcohol on his breath.
B	Shallow with obvious stridor present.
C	Weak, regular radial pulses, capillary refill normal.
Wet Check	Kris is not wearing a shirt and is wet from being dumped with water after he was burned.
CC	Burns with associated dyspnea.

History

S	Obvious burns to the patient's face, chest, abdomen, arms, and hands.
A	Aspirin.
M	Antabuse (has not been taking, discontinued one week ago).
P	Bystanders advise your partner that Kris has a "drinking problem."
L	BBQ hotdogs at approximately 18:00hrs.
E	It appears that the patient was lighting the bonfire and fell into it while trying to move away from the flames.

Assessment

H/N	Severe burns on the patient's face with blistering on his forehead, eyes, and around his mouth and neck. The patient is unable to open his eyes.
Chest	Obvious first- and second-degree burns on the patient's anterior chest and abdomen. Auscultation reveals bilateral wheezing throughout.
ABD	First-degree burns on the epigastric area and right flank.
Back	Unremarkable.
Pelvis	Unremarkable.
Ext	Blistering and redness on both hands and wrists. You observe that the patient is wearing several rings on his fingers.

Vitals

BP	144/96
P	150
RR	28 shallow
Pupils	Eyes closed
GCS	4+4+6=14
BS	5.1 mmol/l
Pulse oximetry	84%
Skin	Pale, diaphoretic on unaffected areas

Pain Assessment

O	n/a
P	n/a
Q	n/a
R	n/a
S	n/a
T	n/a

Cardiac Monitor

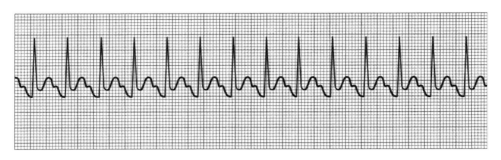

Figure 5.2

Initial Treatment Post Assessment

The patient should be seated on a stretcher to prevent further injuries. Oxygen saturation and administration should be delivered promptly via NRB at 12–15 lpm. Since the patient cannot see, ongoing communication should be continued to inform him of the treatment you will be providing. The burns on the patient's face and neck should be treated with damp dressings. The remainder of the burns on his hands and flank should be treated with wet burn dressings. An IV should be initiated and run at TKVO. An ACP should use analgesics cautiously, as the patient has ingested alcohol. Fentanyl or Morphine Sulphate can be administered to control pain. His rings should be removed and brought to the hospital. Rapid transport of this patient to a burn unit is required.

En route to the hospital, the patient complains of increased pain and moderate dyspnea. There is still adequate air exchange and there are now no signs of obvious stridor or an obstructed airway.

Treatment Continued

Ongoing assessment should continue and dressings should be routinely dampened (if wet) and reapplied. Analgesics can continue to be administered provided the patient is conscious and his respiratory status is adequate.

Differential Diagnosis

- First-, second- and third-degree burns.

Test Your Knowledge

1. What is the total body surface area of the patient's burns?
2. What medication had the patient been prescribed?
3. If the patient had been taking his medication and drinking alcohol, what additional complaints would he have?
4. How do burns in adults differ from burns in children or infants?
5. What is the interpretation of the patient's ECG?

6. What may have caused Kris to fall into the fire?
7. Should the patient's rings be removed? Why?
8. In relation to your patient's burns, what is he at risk of?

CASE 5.3

You are dispatched to Baffin Industrial, 1412 Palugaa St., Iqaluit, for a 26-year-old who may have sustained burns. You are familiar with this address as it is approximately 10 minutes from the Regional Hospital. As you approach the building, you are directed inside, where you see a group of people wiping down a young man. The man's co-workers tell you that Hunter was working with phenol, a caustic, and that the container tipped over, splashing his face, hands, and arms. They took off his shirt and began saturating him with water, without any luck. A co-worker then arrived with alcohol, which helps dissolve the sticky solution. They applied the isopropyl alcohol to Hunter's face and are now applying it to his limbs.

Initial Assessment Findings & Chief Complaint

LOA	Conscious.
A	Patent.
B	Shallow.
C	Strong radial pulse.
Wet Check	Wet with water.
CC	Burn.

History

S	Extreme pain in face, lower arms, and hands.
A	None.
M	None.
P	Healthy.
L	Breakfast.
E	Hunter, the patient, was working with phenol when the container spilled, splashing his face, forearms, and hands. His co-workers removed his shirt and started applying water followed by alcohol to remove the caustic.

Assessment

H/N	Face is wet, mottled red with white areas.
Chest	Unremarkable.
ABD	Small mottled red area just above belt line, with phenol still on abdomen.
Back	Unremarkable.
Pelvis	Stable.
Ext	Entire lower arms and hands are red, with some blisters developing. Distal pulses are present.

Vitals

BP	140/80
P	150, regular
RR	24
Pupils	PERL 4+ mm
GCS	4+5+6=15
BS	n/a
Pulse oximetry	100%
Skin	Wet, warm to touch

Pain Assessment

O	Sudden
P	Industrial accident
Q	Burning
R	Affected area
S	10/10
T	20 minutes

Cardiac Monitor

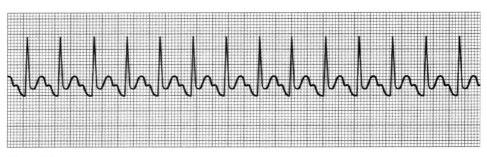

Figure 5.3

Initial Treatment Post Assessment

Initial treatment should include an assessment of the ABCs. With the help of the patient's co-workers, the remainder of the phenol should be removed and irrigated with water. A thorough assessment should then be completed to ensure all phenol is eliminated. The patient's pants and underwear should be removed, as the phenol at the belt line suggests that it may have reached the groin, and, after cleaning, redness or blistering may be exposed. Oxygen should be administered and a complete set of vitals obtained. An intravenous should be secured and infused at TKVO. An ACP should administer narcotic analgesics according to protocol. Rapid transport to a hospital should be initiated. The burns should be covered with damp dressings and saturated en route with sterile water or NS.

En route, the patient complains of increased difficulty breathing and pain. The hospital is now just two minutes away, and the patient has remained awake throughout.

Treatment Continued

The burn dressings should continue to be irrigated with water as long as the patient does not show signs of hypothermia. Airway and breathing assessment are paramount because of the burns on the patient's face. IV analgesics should continue to be administered en route, post vitals assessment.

Differential Diagnosis

- Phenol burns of the first-, second-, and third-degree.

Test Your Knowledge

1. What is significant about the treatment Hunter is receiving as you arrive on scene?
2. What is the most important task at hand when you arrive?
3. What is phenol?
4. What else can be used to aid in the removal of phenol?
5. If the phenol is not removed with alcohol, what could happen to the burns?
6. Based on the description, what type of burns did Hunter sustain?
7. What ECG does the patient present with?
8. How would burns of this degree typically be treated?

Answers
Case 5.1

1. *Using the "Rule of Nines," what is the approximate total burned body surface area on this patient?*

Upper chest	4.5%
Lower chest	4.5%
Abdomen	4.5%
Anterior neck	2.0%
Anterior arms	4.0% (2% each)
Total BSA:	19.5%

2. *Describe the pathology of shock in burn patients.*

   Usually within 24–26 hours, fluid shifts from the vascular compartments to interstitial areas. This results in edema formation and hypovolemia, resulting in hypotension and a sympathetic response.

3. *Would this patient's burns be considered major, moderate or minor?*

   This patient's burns would be considered major or critical. Any third-degree burn in a child warrants this classification.

4. *Why was compliance poor while ventilating this child?*

   Compliance was poor while ventilating this child due to acute respiratory distress that may have developed from inhalation injuries and burns on her face and chest. There has been fluid leakage across the alveolocapillary membrane, resulting in non-cardiogenic pulmonary edema.

5. *Why would you not want to cool a second-degree burn that is more extensive than 10–15%?*

   Cooling a major (third-degree) burn in a child may cause hypothermia and escalate burn shock. If cooling is initiated because of varying degrees of burns and you are in proximity to a medical centre, the wet dressing should be covered by a dry dressing, which would limit cooling. The patient should be kept warm with blankets. If shivering develops, cooling efforts should be discontinued.

6. *Upon arrival at the hospital, fluid resuscitation should be initiated. Using the Parkland Burn Formula, how much fluid should be infused over a 24-hour period?*

   4 ml/kg / Total BSA = x
   4 ml × (10 y/o × 2 +10) / 19.5%

4ml × 30 kg × 19.5 = 2340 ml
2340 ml / 2 = 1170 ml

The patient would receive 1170 ml of fluid (normal saline or Lactated Ringer's) in the first eight hours and the remainder over the following 16 hours.

7. *What classification of medications is the patient on?*

   Theophylline (Aminophylline) – Bronchodilator
   Tegretol (carbamazepine)   – Anticonvulsant, antimanic

8. *What ECG does the patient present with?*

   The patient is presenting in a sinus tachycardia.

Case 5.2

1. *What is the total body surface area of the patient's burns?*

Head:	4.5%
Neck:	1.0%
Chest/ABD:	18.0%
Flank:	3.0%
Hands:	2.0%
Total BSA:	28.5%

2. *What medication had the patient been prescribed?*

   Antabuse (disulfiram) – Alcohol antagonist

3. *If the patient had been taking his medication and drinking alcohol, what additional complaints would he have?*

   This medication is used in conjunction with counselling and support to treat alcoholism. Antabuse works by blocking the processing of alcohol in the body. If alcohol is ingested, the patient may have reactions such as flushing, throbbing headache, tachypnea, nausea, vomiting, dizziness, extreme tiredness, fainting, and a fast or irregular heartbeat. More serious reactions to this medication mixed with alcohol may include seizures and loss of consciousness.

4. *How do burns in adults differ from burns in children or infants?*

	Adult	Child	Infant
Head	9	15	20
Chest	18	15	13
Back	18	15	13
Arms	9 × 2	10 × 2	10 × 2
Legs	18 × 2	15 × 2	14 × 2
Genitals	1	1	1
Buttocks	2 × 2	1.5 × 2	

5. *What is the interpretation of this patient's ECG?*

   The patient is presenting in a sinus tachycardia.

6. *What may have caused Kris to fall into the fire?*

   Kris may have fallen into the fire because of his consumption of alcohol and the resulting unsteadiness.

7. *Should the patient's rings be removed? Why?*

   Rings may impede circulation and should be removed to prevent edema forming distally.

8. *In relation to your patient's burns, what is he at risk of?*

   Kris is at risk of having an obstructed airway as a result of the burns on his face and neck. Edema formation can cause laryngeal edema and airway obstruction. The presence of stridor should be a warning sign. As with all burns, sepsis is also a concern.

Case 5.3

1. *What is significant about the treatment Hunter is receiving as you arrive on scene?*

   The patient is being irrigated with water and his colleagues are removing phenol with the use of alcohol. By removing the phenol, they are stopping the burning process. This is significant, as the burning would continue otherwise.

2. *What is the most important task at hand when you arrive?*

   The most important task when you arrive is the continuation of the removal of phenol, halting of the burning process, and assessing the patient. Because of the burns on his face, you must also be concerned with the potential of airway occlusion due to swelling.

3. *What is phenol?*

   Phenol (carbolic acid) is a corrosive organic acid used widely in industry and medicine. It has an unpleasant odour. Although phenol is diluted commercially, a concentration of even 1–2% may cause burns if in contact with bare skin. Compounds chemically related to phenol include creosol, creosote, and cresylic acid.

4. *What else can be used to aid in the removal of phenol?*

   Phenol can also be removed using a mixture of polyethylene glycol and industrial methylated spirits. This will not only reduce the extent of cutaneous corrosion but also decrease systemic toxicity. Glycerol and the use of an isopropyl alcohol rinse may be superior to water alone in removing phenol.

5. *If the phenol is not removed with alcohol, what may happen to the burns?*

   If the phenol is not removed, coagulation necrosis of the involved area is common. Necrotic tissue may temporarily delay absorption, but phenol could become trapped under the eschar.

6. *Based on the description, what type of burns did Hunter sustain?*

   Hunter sustained the following burns:

Face:	Second- and third-degree burns	4.5%
Arms:	First-, second-, and third-degree burns	9.0%
Genitalia:	First- and second-degree burns	1.0%
Abdomen:	First-degree burns	1.0%
Total BSA		15.5%

7. *What ECG does the patient present with?*

   The patient is presenting in a sinus tachycardia.

8. *How would burns of this degree typically be treated?*

   First- and second-degree burns are treated with damp/wet dressings, and third-degree burns should be treated with dry dressings. Because of the close proximity to the hospital and the cause of the burns, damp dressings should be utilized.

Chapter 6
Musculoskeletal Trauma

With the exception of bilateral femur and pelvis fractures, isolated injuries to extremities rarely threaten a patient's life. The presence of such fractures in extremities, however, may suggest other potential fractures or injuries in a patient. The mechanism of injury is important in anticipating potential injuries elsewhere in the body, including simple fractures. With isolated fractures, treatment is therefore usually delayed until a thorough assessment has been completed and other interventions established. The goal in treating isolated musculoskeletal trauma is to stabilize and immobilize the affected limb to prevent further injury and to maintain adequate perfusion. In the presence of a dislocation or fracture immobilization, it is important to ensure that there is limited neurovascular injury. Isolated limb injuries should be assessed for the six Ps: pain, pulselessness, paresthesia, paralysis, pallor, and pressure, both pre- and post-immobilization.

CASE 6.1

At 14:30hrs on a warm summer day, you are dispatched to an accident involving a farm tractor at the O.K. Corral, a farm just outside Chelmsford, Ontario. You are approximately 10 minutes from the scene and another 25 minutes from the receiving hospital. On arrival, you are directed to a large tin building, the size of a small arena, evidently used for horseback riding in the winter. Once inside, you see a tractor in front of the patient, who is lying down. The tractor has been shut off. The ground in the riding arena is beach sand, and even though the weather is warm outside, it is much cooler in the building. The patient, an approximately 50-year-old female, looks pale and is in a fair amount of pain. Her son Kevin, who is on scene, tells you that his mother, Laura, was struck in the upper legs by the bucket of the tractor. She was standing in front of the tractor as he was shutting it down when the clutch jumped, causing the bucket to hit Laura's legs. Laura was knocked to the ground and started crying and complaining of pain in her legs. She has not moved from the point of impact.

Initial Assessment Findings & Chief Complaint

LOA	Conscious and alert.
A	Patent.
B	Regular and full volume at approximately 16.
C	Strong radial pulses.
Wet Check	Small amount of blood through the patient's jeans at mid-thigh bilaterally.
CC	Possible fractured legs.

History

S	Patient is complaining of pain in bilateral upper legs.
A	None.
M	HCT, Fosamax, Evista, Slow-K.
P	Osteoporosis, hypertension, cholecystectomy 10 years ago.
L	Lunch at 12:30hrs.
E	The patient was struck in the mid-thigh by the bucket of a tractor and knocked to the ground. There was no loss of consciousness. The patient complains of feeling pins and needles in both lower legs.

Assessment

H/N	Unremarkable, no JVD, trachea midline, no c-spine pain.
Chest	Unremarkable, equal air entry bilaterally.
ABD	Soft/non-tender, mid-line surgical scar.
Back	Unremarkable and no pain on palpation.
Pelvis	Stable.
Ext	Upper extremities are unremarkable, while bilateral lower extremities have an abrasion mid-thigh and pain on palpation with obvious instability. Capillary refill and distal circulation are present.

Vitals

BP	92/68
P	150, regular
RR	16 full volume
Pupils	PERL 4+ mm
GCS	4+5+6=15
BS	n/a
Pulse oximetry	98%
Skin	Pale, diaphoretic

Pain Assessment

O	n/a
P	n/a
Q	n/a
R	n/a
S	n/a
T	n/a

Cardiac Monitor

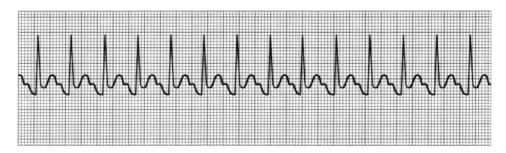

Figure 6.1

Initial Treatment Post Assessment

Initial treatment should include manual c-spine stabilization until a possible spinal injury can be ruled out. A complete assessment should be performed, including sensation and circulation distal to the suspected fractures. Supplemental oxygen should be administered and a complete set of vitals and ECG interpretation obtained. In this case, spinal immobilization can be ruled out as the patient was knocked to the ground and there was no impact involving c-spine. The patient was knocked from a standing position onto beach sand. A traction splint should be applied to the bilateral femurs as they both appear to be closed, with external superficial abrasions caused by the bucket of the tractor. Traction in the amount of 20% of the patient's body weight (to a maximum of 30 lb traction) should be applied to the splint. Post application of traction, assessment of the distal extremities should be completed. The patient can then be transferred to a stretcher via a fracture board or scoop stretcher to reduce the risk of movement and pain. The patient should be placed in a position of comfort. An intravenous should be initiated and a 20 ml/kg bolus started in order to sustain a BP of 100/P.

En route to the hospital, the patient's BP is 108/68 and her pulse is 100 bpm after a 500 ml bolus of normal saline. There are large ecchymoses present in both anterior thighs.

Treatment Continued

The bolus should be discontinued and the IV infused at TKVO. Further assessment of the lower extremities should be performed to ensure adequate circulation is present.

Differential Diagnosis

- Bilateral fractured femurs.

Test Your Knowledge

1. What is the basis for ruling out c-spine precautions on this patient?
2. What classifications are your patient's medications?
3. What is the patient's ECG rhythm?
4. Approximately how much blood loss is possible with a bilateral femur fracture?
5. What is the rationale for applying a traction splint?
6. What medical condition would make the patient more susceptible to fractures?
7. Why would this patient not be a candidate for IV analgesics?
8. What is a contraindication for utilizing a traction splint?
9. What should you do if, after applying a traction splint, you cannot find a distal pulse (dorsalis pedis)?

CASE 6.2

You are dispatched at 10:30hrs to a property close to South Indian Lake, Manitoba, for a possible drilling accident. On arrival, you are met by the site foreman who tells you that Andre, a 40-year-old employee, got his arm stuck in a core sampler drill. Apparently, a piece of his clothing was caught, which pulled his arm into the drill and twisted it around the drill bit. As Andre pulled free of the machine, he fell six metres from a platform. He is now lying prone at the base of the platform. A few of his colleagues are crouched beside him. You notice an obvious angulation of his left leg and that his left arm is tucked under him. As you introduce yourself, he tells you that he feels as though his arm has been torn off.

Initial Assessment Findings & Chief Complaint

LOA	Conscious but confused.
A	Patent.
B	Spontaneous.
C	Strong radial pulse (right only).
Wet Check	No obvious bleeding noted.
CC	Musculoskeletal trauma.

History

S	Pain in his leg, back, and arm.
A	None.
M	glyburide, Atasol-30.
P	NIDDM, sciatica.
L	Breakfast.
E	The patient was working on a drilling platform when his arm was caught in the bit. As he tried to free himself, he fell from a platform to the ground. There was no loss of consciousness, but he was unable to get up and is in severe pain.

Assessment

H/N	Small abrasion on the patient's forehead.
Chest	Unremarkable with equal air entry bilaterally.
ABD	Soft/non-tender.
Back	No obvious trauma noted, but the patient has pain in the lower lumbar region.
Pelvis	Stable.
Ext	Right upper and lower extremities unremarkable, left lower leg angulated laterally, and upper arm torsion injury with bone twisted and exposed. The wrist appears mangled and white. No radial pulse is present in the left arm, which is white, with blood on the forearm.

Vitals

BP	100/60
P	150, regular
RR	20
Pupils	PERL 4+ mm
GCS	4+4+6=14
BS	4.1 mmol/l
Pulse oximetry	96%
Skin	Pale, diaphoretic

Pain Assessment

O	At time of fall
P	Trauma
Q	Constant
R	None
S	10/10
T	30 minutes

Cardiac Monitor

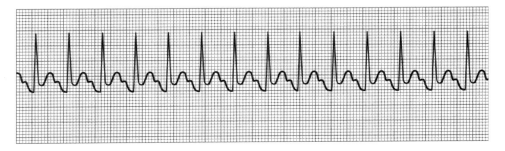

Figure 6.2

Initial Treatment Post Assessment

Initial treatment should include manual c-spine immobilization while an assessment is performed. Once the patient has been log-rolled to a fracture board, assessment should continue. A baseline set of vitals should be obtained including blood glucometry and SPO2. The patient should be administered oxygen via a high concentration mask. A cervical collar should be applied and the patient secured to the board. The patient's leg should then be assessed for distal circulation. His torsion arm should be covered with a sterile dressing and splinted as best as possible in an attempt to immobilize it. The patient should then be packaged promptly and readied for transport. Cardiac monitoring should be initiated. Once en route to the hospital, an intravenous should be initiated and infused at TKVO.

En route, the patient complains of more pain in the lower leg. He is nauseated and complains of being dizzy.

Treatment Continued

Reassessment of the extremities and vitals should be performed. An ACP should administer narcotic analgesics such as morphine or fentanyl as long as the patient's vitals remain stable. Rapid transport to a trauma centre should not be delayed.

Differential Diagnosis

- Femur fracture.
- Torsion injury in forearm.

Test Your Knowledge

1. What injuries might you suspect from the patient's fall?
2. What are typical signs of poor circulation in the patient's injured arm?
3. What is sciatica?
4. What classifications are the patient's medications?
5. What ECG does the patient present with?
6. What are the classifications of musculoskeletal injuries, and what category would Andre's injuries be listed in?

Answers

Case 6.1

1. *What is the basis for ruling out c-spine precautions on this patient?*
   The patient was struck only in the legs, causing her to fall onto a soft surface (beach sand) without striking her back or head. Regardless of her history of osteoporosis, the mechanism of injury does not dictate spinal immobilization.

2. **What classifications are your patient's medications?**

HCT (hydrochlorothiazide)	– Diuretic
Fosamax (alendronate)	– Inhibits osteoclast
Evista (raloxifene)	– Estrogen receptor modulator
Slow-K (potassium)	– Potassium supplement

3. **What is the patient's ECG rhythm?**

   The patient is presenting in a sinus tachycardia.

4. **Approximately how much blood loss is possible with a bilateral femur fracture?**

   The patient can lose up to and including one litre from each fractured femur, which in some people could amount to 40% of their circulating blood volume.

5. **What is the rationale for applying a traction splint?**

   When a femur is fractured, and because of the crisscross fashion of the thigh muscles, the normally cylindrical thigh becomes spherical. The potential area of thigh is now increased, and bleeding ensues, adding more volume to the space. This increases the amount of pressure at the injury site, which may lead to increased pain and spasms. The expectation of the traction splint is that it will apply specific tension to the leg allowing it to regain its cylindrical shape, therefore reducing pressure and pain. This device is ideally applied to patients who are experiencing muscle spasms. Once the initial traction is applied, it should not be reapplied. As the leg relaxes, it will need less traction to maintain its normal pre-injury shape.

6. **What medical condition would make the patient more susceptible to fractures?**

   The patient has a history of osteoporosis, a condition in which bone density is reduced. The typical bone microarchitecture is disrupted and the number and variety of non-collagenous proteins within the bone are altered.

7. **Why would this patient not be a candidate for IV analgesics?**

   The patient would not be a candidate for IV analgesics, particularly morphine or fentanyl, because of her low blood pressure. At this time, the patient is hypotensive with a compensatory heart rate.

8. **What is a contraindication for utilizing a traction splint?**

   One contraindication for the use of a traction splint is a pelvic fracture.

9. **What should you do if, after applying a traction splint, you cannot find a distal pulse (dorsalis pedis)?**

   If the traction splint is applied and a distal pulse is not longer palpable, the traction should be removed in increments until distal circulation returns.

Case 6.2

1. **What injuries might you suspect from the patient's fall?**

   Based on the mechanism of injury and the distance fallen, the patient could potentially have numerous injuries, including the following:

   Obvious torsion injury in arm
   Possible fracture in injured leg
   Possible head trauma
   Possible cervical/back injury
   Possible internal injuries
   Query associated medical injuries

2. **What are typical signs of poor circulation in the patient's injured arm?**

   Signs and symptoms of poor circulation in the patient's injured arm may include the following:
   - Poor colour
   - Paresthesia
   - Paralysis
   - Absence of pulse
   - Pain

3. **What is sciatica?**

   Sciatica is severe pain along the course of the sciatic nerve, usually felt at the back of the thigh and running down the leg. Common causes of sciatica include disk herniation, intraspinal tumor, foraminal stenosis, extraspinal plexus compression, piriformis syndrome, and spinal stenosis.

4. **What classifications are the patient's medications?**

Medication	Classification
glyburide (Diabeta)	Oral hypoglycemic
Atasol-30 (Acetaminophen with codeine)	Narcotic analgesic

5. **What ECG does the patient present with?**

   The patient is presenting with a sinus tachycardia.

6. **What are the classifications of musculoskeletal injuries, and what category would Andre's injuries be listed in?**

   The classifications of musculoskeletal injuries include the following:
   - Life- and limb-threatening injuries
   - Life-threatening injuries, minor musculoskeletal injuries
   - Non life-threatening injuries, serious limb-threatening injuries
   - Non life-threatening injuries, isolated minor musculoskeletal injuries

   The patient is presenting with a life- and limb-threatening injury

Chapter 7
Face, Head, and Neck Trauma

The head, face, and neck are essential structures for life, and their continuity is so important that their immobilization is paramount upon arrival at an injury scene. Manual stabilization of the neck and head should be initiated any time a mechanism of injury dictates potential compromise to these areas. The patient's mentation should be assessed and routinely re-evaluated throughout transport to a hospital to ensure cerebral perfusion. Full immobilization should occur on patients suspected of a possible head/neck/spinal injury. Oxygenation should also be provided, and unconscious patients should be ventilated to provide perfusion and limit the increase of intracranial pressure. Ongoing communication with the patient should serve to reassess potential of life-altering injuries.

CASE 7.1

At 17:35hrs on a clear summer day, you are dispatched to a single vehicle accident on Highway 1 near Cavendish, Prince Edward Island. On arrival, you observe that police and volunteer firefighters are on scene. A firefighter approaches and reports that a female of approximately 16 years was thrown from her car into a ditch after the car had rolled several times. He tells you that the patient is conscious but not making any sense. As you approach, you see another firefighter maintaining c-spine support while the patient lies supine in the ditch. You ask the patient's name and she tries to talk, making a long, drawn-out attempt, but you can't understand her. The patient looks at you with confusion.

Initial Assessment Findings & Chief Complaint

LOA	Semi-conscious.
A	Patent.
B	Regular, full volume.
C	Strong radial pulses.
Wet Check	Bleeding from nose, lacerations on upper lip and side of mouth.
CC	Trauma.

History

S	Confused as to surroundings.
A	CNO.
M	CNO.
P	CNO.
L	CNO.
E	The patient was the apparent driver of a vehicle that rolled several times and landed in a ditch. She was thrown from the vehicle.

Assessment

H/N	Possible fractured nose, with dried blood on both nostrils. Edema of the right eye (closed), superior to the forehead and laterally to the right occipital lobe. Bruising present under right eye. Laceration present on the left corner of the mouth and upper lip. Teeth appear intact.
Chest	Symmetrical, unremarkable, equal air entry bilaterally.
ABD	Unremarkable.
Back	7-cm abrasion on right buttock.
Pelvis	Stable.
Ext	Swelling and discolouration on left foot and lower leg. Bilateral mobility of upper and lower extremities with normal capillary refill and distal pulses. Edema and abrasions on the left wrist.

Vitals

BP	100/60
P	75, regular
RR	14 full volume
Pupils	L: PERL 3+ mm
	R: eye closed (swollen)
GCS	3+3+4=10
BS	6.3 mmol/l
Pulse oximetry	97%
Skin	Pale, warm

Pain Assessment

O	n/a
P	n/a
Q	n/a
R	n/a
S	n/a
T	n/a

Cardiac Monitor

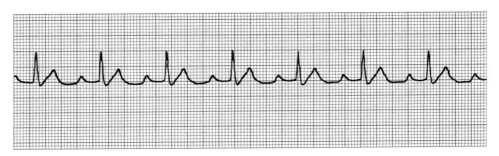

Figure 7.1

Initial Treatment Post Assessment

The patient should continue to have c-spine support while an assessment is performed. Oxygen should be administered with a high concentration mask. After assessment, a complete set of vitals should be obtained. A cervical collar should be applied and the patient immobilized on a fracture board. Rapid transport should be a priority. En route to the hospital, cardiac monitoring should be performed. An intravenous should be initiated and run at TKVO. Dressings can be applied to various lacerations/abrasions. ACP and PCP have the same specifics in treatment for this patient.

En route, the patient becomes more confused and begins mumbling. She is very restless and is trying to wiggle off the fracture board.

Treatment Continued

Current supportive care should be continued, ensuring that the patient is oxygenated en route to the hospital. The patient may have to be restrained in order to maintain immobilization. Carefully monitor vital signs and GCS every five minutes.

Differential Diagnosis

- Closed head injury.
- Possible subdural hematoma.

Test Your Knowledge

1. What is significant about the patient's position when you arrive on scene?
2. Based on the mechanism of injury, what injuries might you have anticipated from this accident?
3. What are the typical signs and symptoms of a closed head injury due to trauma?
4. How should a patient with a head injury be treated on scene?
5. What are the common causes of subdural hematoma?
6. What ECG is the patient presenting with?
7. What are the two phases of acute brain injuries and how do they differ?
8. What best describes diffuse axonal injury?

CASE 7.2

At 03:00hrs, you are dispatched to Campus de Val-d'Or at the Université du Québec for a patient who has been found outside. On arrival, you are greeted by a group of students who tell you that they have found a guy who looks as though he has been beaten up. They report that he is lying behind a residence. As approach the patient, you notice droplets of blood on the sidewalk. You observe a young male, probably 16 or 17 years old, lying on his stomach. As you near, he makes no effort to communicate verbally. You ask your partner to maintain c-spine support as you begin assessment. Just as you reach the patient's side, the police and fire department arrive on scene.

Initial Assessment Findings & Chief Complaint

LOA	Responsive to painful stimuli, with decorticate posturing.
A	Patent.
B	Shallow and slow.
C	Radial pulse present, irregular.
Wet Check	Blood on face, neck, hands, and incontinent of urine and feces.
CC	Possible assault.

History

S	The patient was possibly assaulted and was found by passersby.
A	MedicAlert tag: penicillin.
M	CNO.
P	CNO.
L	CNO.
E	No information regarding who the patient is or how he came to be at the residence.

Assessment

H/N	Dried blood on both nares, multiple abrasions on left side of face, swelling of the occipital and left parietal areas, and a possible break in the continuity of the skull.
Chest	Multiple abrasions on the left chest with possible rib fractures. Equal air entry bilaterally.
ABD	Firm, rigid with abrasions.
Back	Unremarkable.
Pelvis	Stable.
Ext	Multiple abrasions on both hands. Decorticate posturing during assessment of the patient.

Vitals

BP	190/100
P	45
RR	8 shallow
Pupils	PERL 5 mm, slow to react
GCS	1+2+3=6
BS	5.8 mmol/l
Pulse oximetry	84%
Skin	Pale, cool

Pain Assessment

O	n/a
P	n/a
Q	n/a
R	n/a
S	n/a
T	n/a

Cardiac Monitor

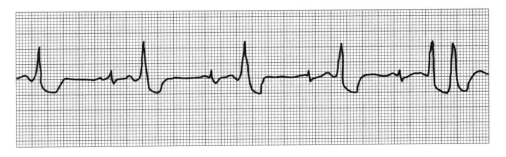

Figure 7.2

Initial Treatment Post Assessment

The additional resources of the fire department can be utilized to help immobilize the patient's c-spine. His airway should be assessed and suctioned if required. An OPA should be inserted (if tolerated) and the patient hyperventilated with a BVM and oxygen at 20–24 breaths per minute. A thorough assessment should be performed and the patient placed and secured on a fracture board. Transport to an emergency facility should be prompt. An intravenous should be initiated en route. An ACP should initiate endotrachial intubation and confirm its placement.

En route, the patient's vital signs are BP 200/90, P 40, RR 6 (assisted at 20), with warm skin.

Treatment Continued

The patient should be reassessed routinely throughout transport, and manual patient ventilation should be continued en route. Assessment of vital signs should be ongoing.

Differential Diagnosis

- Head injury with increased ICP.

Test Your Knowledge

1. Based on the patient's presentation, what do you think happened to him?
2. What may be the signs and symptoms of Cushing's reflex?
3. What are the signs and symptoms of brain injury?
4. How is Central Syndrome best described?
5. Why might the patient have bilaterally dilated pupils?
6. What facial feature should be observed carefully when assessing and reassessing a head injury patient?
7. What ECG rhythm is the patient presenting with?
8. What cyclic breathing pattern may be seen with a severe head injury?

Answers

Case 7.1

1. *What is significant about the patient's position when you arrive on scene?*

   Based on the patient's location, it would appear that she was thrown a considerable distance from the vehicle.

2. *Based on the mechanism of injury, what injuries might you have anticipated from this accident?*

   The possibility of death or multiple traumas might be anticipated by the mechanism of injury. Head and spinal injuries are common in patients ejected from vehicles during accidents. Chest, pelvic, and internal injuries should also be anticipated.

3. *What are the typical signs and symptoms of a closed head injury due to trauma?*

   Typical signs of a head injury vary depending on the extent of injury and its location in the skull. Such injuries will usually present with an altered level of consciousness or a state of unconsciousness. Vital signs may also vary, but can present as normotensive and may progress to increased blood pressure and decreased heart rate and respiratory rate if there is an increase in ICP.

4. *How should a patient with a head injury be treated on a scene?*

   A patient with a suspected head injury should be presumed to have a neck injury and should have complete spinal immobilization with a c-collar and fracture board. Administer oxygen and assist with the patient's ventilation if required. Hyperventilate if the patient is exhibiting signs of cerebral herniation, as evidenced by a deteriorating GCS or other signs and symptoms.

5. *What are the common causes of subdural hematoma?*

   Common causes of subdural hematoma vary based on whether the hematoma is chronic or acute. Acute injuries include those caused by sudden acceleration and deceleration of the brain parenchyma and tearing of the bridging veins. The onset of acute symptoms develops within 14 days. Chronic injuries may present in alcoholics or the elderly, who may report changes in levels of awareness or less specific complaints.

6. *What ECG is the patient presenting with?*

   The patient is presenting in a first-degree AV block.

7. *What are the two phases of acute brain injuries and how do they differ?*

   Acute brain injuries include primary and secondary phases. The primary or acute phase involves the death or cellular injury of the brain as a direct result of the injury. The secondary phase can occur hours to weeks after the injury and can cause temporary and permanent damage to previously unharmed cells. This later injury can be caused by vascular injuries or compressive forces.

8. *What best describes diffuse axonal injury?*

   Diffuse axonal injury is best described as any type of brain injury caused by stretching, shearing, or tearing of nerve fibres.

Case 7.2

1. *Based on the patient's presentation, what do you think happened to him?*

   Based on the presentation of the patient, he was possibly assaulted and may have sustained chest, head, and abdominal injuries.

2. *What may be the signs and symptoms of Cushing's reflex?*

   Cushing's reflex includes an increase in blood pressure and falling respiratory and heart rates.

3. *What are the signs and symptoms of brain injury?*

   Some typical signs and symptoms of brain injury may include:

   Confusion or altered level of consciousness
   Disorientation
   Personality change
   Amnesia
   Cushing's reflex
   Vomiting
   Body temperature fluctuations
   Changes in pupil reactivity
   Decorticate or decerebrate posturing

4. *How is Central Syndrome best described?*

   Central Syndrome is an upper brainstem compression that produces an increase in blood pressure to maintain cerebral perfusion pressure (CPP) and a reflex decrease in heart rate in response to the vagus nerve stimulation of the SA and AV nodes.

5. *Why might the patient have bilaterally dilated pupils?*

   The patient's pupils may be dilated because of increasing ICP pressing on the oculomotor nerve (cranial nerve III).

6. *What facial feature should be observed carefully when assessing and reassessing a head injury patient?*

   Pay close attention to the eyes when assessing and reassessing patients suffering from head injuries. Eyes can indicate possible problems with cranial nerves II, III, IV, and VI.

7. *What ECG rhythm is the patient presenting with?*

   The patient is presenting in a Normal Sinus Rhythm (NSR) with premature ventricular contractions (PVCs).

8. *What cyclic breathing pattern may be seen with a severe head injury?*

   Cheyne-Stokes respiration may be seen with a severe head injury, which is evidenced by increasing and then decreasing respiration volumes.

Chapter 8
Spinal Trauma

Spinal injury is frequently associated with trauma-related accidents, such as falls, motor-vehicle collisions, sports injuries, and other contact incidents. The possible results of spinal trauma are death or permanent disability. Spinal precautions should be taken with all patients who have a reduced level of consciousness or when the mechanism of injury has the potential to cause a spinal injury. Common injuries associated with trauma to the spinal column include column injury, cord injury, spinal shock, neurogenic shock, and autonomic hyperreflexia syndrome. As well as physical injuries, emotional or psychological injuries warrant ongoing communication and support. Pre-hospital care of a potential spinal injury may make a significant difference in the patient's long-term level of mobility.

CASE 8.1

You are dispatched to the Cape Breton Highlands National Park at 14:45hrs for a possible motocross accident. On arrival, you are met by two hikers, Cathy and Leena, and directed to a small valley where you observe an overturned motocross bike. Approximately five metres away, the patient is lying prone in a ditch. As you approach, you hear him calling for help. He appears alert and oriented to your presence and tells you that his name is Dan and he is 18 years old. Once at his side, your partner maintains c-spine support and you begin your assessment. The patient is wearing a helmet, which does not appear to have sustained any damage. He tells you he hit a tree stump while riding and his motocross bike flew into the air. He was thrown from the bike, landing on his face. He has not been able to move since. He is not sure of the time but thinks he has been lying on the ground for quite a while.

Initial Assessment Findings & Chief Complaint

LOA	Oriented as to the incident and surroundings.
A	Appears patent.
B	Normal at approximately 16.
C	Strong radial pulses.
Wet Check	Incontinent of urine and feces.
CC	Possible spinal injury.

History

S	Complains of not being able to move, no presence of pain.
A	None.
M	Unknown medication for acne.
P	None.
L	Breakfast.
E	The patient was riding his motocross bike at approximately 50 km/hr when he hit a tree stump, forcing his bike into the air. He was thrown from the bike and landed in a ditch. He does not think he lost consciousness as he remembers the entire incident.

Assessment

H/N	Unremarkable without obvious trauma. No JVD, trachea midline, alcohol detected on the patient's breath.
Chest	Symmetrical with equal air entry bilaterally.
ABD	Soft, flaccid.
Back	No obvious trauma noted. The patient is able to feel your touch to his occipital area, but loses sensation to palpation in the lower neck.
Pelvis	Stable.
Ext	Complete paralysis of body and lower extremities. Upper extremities reveal minor wrist extension and elbow flexion. The patient appears to have an erection.

Vitals

BP	110/60
P	75 strong and regular
RR	16 full volume
Pupils	PERL 4+ mm
GCS	4+5+6=15
BS	n/a
Pulse oximetry	98%
Skin	Warm, dry

Pain Assessment

O	n/a
P	n/a
Q	n/a
R	n/a
S	n/a
T	n/a

Cardiac Monitor

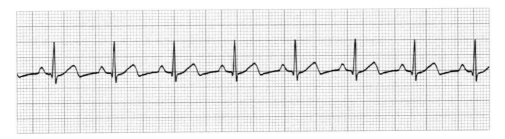

Figure 8.1

Initial Treatment Post Assessment

C-spine control should be maintained by your partner as you perform a primary assessment. Airway patency must be ensured and oxygen administered via a high concentration mask. With the help of the bystanders, the patient should be log-rolled onto a fracture board. His helmet should be removed and a cervical collar applied. The patient should be securely fastened to the fracture board with his head taped in place. A cardiac monitor should be attached and an ECG interpreted. The patient should be transported promptly to an emergency facility. En route, an intravenous should be established and run at TKVO.

During transport, the patient's blood pressure begins to drop and is 88/68. His ECG is a sinus tachycardia at 110. His respiratory rate and oxygen saturation stay constant.

Treatment Continued

Post vitals assessment, the intravenous rate should be increased and a 20 ml/kg bolus administered to sustain a systolic pressure of 100. A continuous airway assessment should continue as the patient may not be able to clear secretions and is at risk of aspiration if he vomits.

Differential Diagnosis

- Possible C6 fracture.

Test Your Knowledge

1. What type of spinal injury is suspected, based on Dan's presentation?
2. Would the presence of alcohol intensify his lack of motor skills?
3. Why is your patient's breathing not affected, given the suspected cervical spine injury?
4. Why is the patient presenting with warm extremities?
5. What ECG is Dan presenting with?
6. Why is Dan's blood pressure decreasing en route to the hospital?
7. What type of assistance will your patient probably require with permanent cord injury at this level?
8. Should Dan's helmet be removed for transport?
9. Why is Dan presenting with what appears to be an erection?

CASE 8.2

At 03:00hrs on a hot August afternoon, you are dispatched to a large party at 1247 Temperance Street, Saskatoon, where someone has fallen into the pool. You, having more seniority, jokingly tell your rookie partner he is going swimming. As you turn onto the street, you see about 40 parked cars and an outpouring of partygoers. You advise dispatch to send police assistance and head to the backyard. As you manoeuvre around the patrons, you see a young woman floating in the pool with support from a few friends. A passerby tells you that Karly, who has had too much to drink, jumped off the roof into the pool, landing hard on her feet in the shallow end. She floated up, saying that her back was sore and she couldn't move.

Initial Assessment Findings & Chief Complaint

LOA	Conscious and alert.
A	Patent.
B	Spontaneous respirations.
C	Strong radial pulses.
Wet Check	Wet, in a pool.
CC	Numbness in lower extremities.

History

S	Anxious and can't get out of the pool.
A	None.
M	Ortho Tri-Cyclen, Cipro.
P	Recent infection.
L	BBQ at the party.
E	Karly was drinking coolers at the party. A group of friends decided to jump from the roof into the pool and she decided to join them, but jumped into the shallow end. She hit the bottom hard with straight legs, and then drifted around in the pool. Others jumped in and supported her as she floated and one friend called 911.

Assessment

H/N	Unremarkable.
Chest	Unremarkable, equal air entry bilaterally.
ABD	Unremarkable.
Back	Pain on palpation in the lower lumbar region, approximately L1/L2.
Pelvis	Stable.
Ext	Good strength, mobility, and range of motion (ROM) in upper extremities. Minimal movement at hips and inability to move legs below the knees. Obvious deformity to bilateral heels.

Vitals

BP	100/60
P	75 strong/regular
RR	14 full volume
Pupils	PERL 5+ mm
GCS	4+5+6=15
BS	n/a
Pulse oximetry	99%
Skin	Warm, normal

Pain Assessment

O	n/a
P	n/a
Q	n/a
R	n/a
S	n/a
T	n/a

Cardiac Monitor

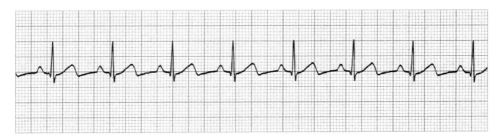

Figure 8.2

Initial Treatment Post Assessment

Initial assessment of the patient should begin in the pool while c-spine is being maintained. The patient should be removed from the pool with a spinal board. Once on the deck, the patient should be kept warm. A c-collar should be applied, and the patient fully immobilized on the spinal board. A complete set of vitals, including SPO2 and cardiac monitoring, should be obtained. A more thorough neurological exam can be completed en route to the hospital. An intravenous infusing at TKVO can be initiated.

Differential Diagnosis

- Spinal cord trauma at L2.
- Bilateral os calis (heel) fractures.

Test Your Knowledge

1. What is significant about the patient's position when you arrive on scene?
2. What ECG rhythm does the patient present with?
3. Based on the patient's movement of her upper extremities and the straightening of her knees, at what level do you anticipate a spinal cord injury?
4. With probable bilateral os calis fractures, what other injuries might you suspect?
5. Should the patient's respiratory status be affected, given that a spinal fracture is suspected?
6. What classifications are the patient's medications?
7. In reference to tools for assessment, what is the most important aspect of scene assessment in this case?

Answers

Case 8.1

1. *What type of spinal injury is suspected, based on Dan's presentation?*

    Based on Dan's mechanism of injury and inability to move his extremities, a c-spine injury should be suspected. Dan is able to breathe on his own and has a weak grip by extending his wrist backward. He has probably injured his cervical spine at C6.

2. *Would the presence of alcohol intensify his lack of motor skills?*

    The presence of alcohol, although a depressant, should not affect the generalized lack of mobility of his upper and lower extremities.

3. *Why is your patient's breathing not affected, given the suspected cervical spine injury?*

    The vertebrae C3, C4, and C5 supply the diaphragm, thereby reinforcing the differential diagnosis of a lower c-spine injury.

4. *Why is the patient presenting with warm extremities?*

    The patient is presenting with warm extremities and skin below the level of injury because of venodilation and vasodilation. The patient will present primarily with cool, moist, and pale skin above the level of injury, and warm, flushed, and dry skin below.

5. *What ECG does Dan present with?*

   The patient is presenting with a normal sinus rhythm.

6. *Why is Dan's blood pressure decreasing en route to the hospital?*

   The patient may be progressing to spinal or neurogenic shock, which occurs when the brain's signals to control the body are interrupted. Vasoconstriction is limited particularly below the level of injury, and therefore the lack of sympathetic tone causes veins and arteries to dilate. As they dilate, they enlarge the body's bucket size (vascular space), causing hypovolemia.

7. *What type of assistance will your patient probably require with permanent cord injury at this level?*

   The patient will require an electric wheelchair for transportation. He will require personal support for feeding, clearing secretions, and meeting his basic everyday needs.

8. *Should Dan's helmet be removed for transport?*

   The patient's helmet should be removed, but not until he is log-rolled onto a fracture board. Once he is supine, and as your partner maintains c-spine control, you should place one hand under the patient's occiput and cradle the jaw and anterior neck with the other. As your partner spreads the helmet and removes it, you should slide your hand to support the occiput superiorly on the back of the head. Once the helmet is off, your partner can then assume c-spine control. The helmet should not be removed while the patient is prone or semi-prone, as adequate support of the head cannot be maintained.

9. *Why is Dan presenting with what appears to be an erection?*

   The patient is presenting with a priapism. This is a prolonged erection of the penis due to unopposed parasympathetic stimulation. In cervical spine injuries, sympathetic pathways can be disrupted and result in this added telltale sign. Although this symptom is not common, one should be suspicious of a spinal injury if the mechanism of injury suggests it.

Case 8.2

1. *What is significant about the patient's position when you arrive on scene?*

   The patient has remained where the injury took place. The water is providing a natural backboard, and, with the support of her friends, she will have positioned herself in neutral alignment. Although extrication may be more difficult for paramedics, the process can be done correctly with minimal injury to the patient.

2. *What ECG rhythm does your patient present with?*

   The patient is presenting in a normal sinus rhythm.

3. *Based on the patient's movement of her upper extremities and the straightening of her knees, at what level do you anticipate a spinal cord injury?*

   The patient is presenting with paralysis of the lower extremities. At the level of L2, the myotones affected are those associated with the bending of the hip, while at L3 the affected muscles are those related to straightening the knee. This patient does have some movement in the hip, but nothing distally. The approximate level of spinal cord injury is therefore L2.

4. *With probable bilateral os calis fractures, what other injuries might you suspect?*

   The patient is presenting with bilateral os calis fractures, which are usually sustained from jumping from a height and landing flat on the feet. She jumped from at least seven metres, landing in the pool. Compression of the lumbar spine would be an expected injury associated with os calis fractures.

5. *Should the patient's respiratory status be affected, given that a spinal fracture is suspected?*

   The patient's respiratory status should not be affected by this spinal injury, as the myotones for respiration and control of the diaphragm are at levels C3, C4, and C5.

6. *What classifications are the patient's medications?*

   Cipro (ciprofloxacin HCl) — Antibiotic
   Ortho Tri-Cyclen (norgestimate and ethinyl estradiol) — Birth control

7. *In reference to tools for assessment, what is the most important aspect of scene assessment in this case?*

   The mechanism of injury will often suggest the possibility of spinal column injury, and a thorough description of what happened is beneficial and will aid in differential diagnosis.

Chapter 9
Thoracic Trauma

Over the past decade, incidences of both blunt and penetrating chest traumas have increased. Blunt trauma is most often related to motor vehicle accidents, and as the number of vehicles on the road increases, so does the incidence of trauma. Penetrating trauma, which has especially increased in urban areas, is related to violent crime. As crime rates rise, so do the rates of penetrating traumas to the chest and abdomen. In assessing these patients, the mechanism of injury and clinical findings will help differentiate potential injuries. Oxygenation should be a priority to increase survival from thoracic trauma. As with all traumas, understanding the potential for internal injuries will assist the paramedic with treatment, particularly with respect to abdominal injuries.

CASE 9.1

At 11:00hrs, you are dispatched to Drayton Valley Ski Hill, Alberta, for a report of an injured snowboarder. You are only a few minutes away but are aware that it will be a long ride to the hospital given the miserable February weather. On your arrival, you are met by a ski patrol member, who tells you that there is a 28-year-old female in the first aid building. He thinks she has sustained a few broken ribs. As you enter the first aid room, you notice that the patient's boots are off and that she is secured to a board and wearing a collar. She is still wearing her ski jacket and clothing. She acknowledges your presence and tells you that the pain is killing her. She tells you that she was coming down the hill and tried to "ride the rail," but fell hard on her left chest.

Initial Assessment Findings & Chief Complaint

LOA	Conscious and alert.
A	Patent.
B	Shallow due to pain.
C	Strong radial pulse.
Wet Check	Unremarkable.
CC	Possible fractured ribs.

History

S	Sore chest.
A	None.
M	Glyburide.
P	NIDDM.
L	Lunch at the ski hill.
E	While attempting to "ride the rail," the patient fell, striking her ribs.

Assessment

H/N	Unremarkable.
Chest	Pain on palpation in left lateral ribs 5, 6, and 7. Equal air entry bilaterally.
ABD	Soft/non-tender.
Back	Unremarkable.
Pelvis	Stable.
Ext	Equal strength and mobility in upper and lower extremities.

Vitals

BP	130/88
P	75, regular
RR	20 shallow
Pupils	PERL 3+ mm
GCS	4+5+6=15
BS	5.1 mmol/l
Pulse oximetry	99%
Skin	Warm and dry

Pain Assessment

O	Sudden
P	Fall
Q	Sharp
R	No radiation
S	10/10
T	25 minutes

Cardiac Monitor

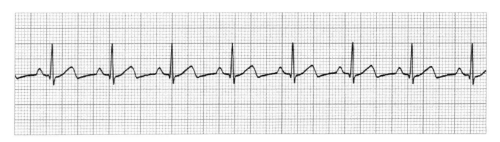

Figure 9.1

Initial Treatment Post Assessment

The patient should be assessed after you attempt to remove her upper clothing and maintain c-spine support. The collar should be reapplied and the patient secured to a fracture board. A complete set of vitals should be obtained, including a blood glucometry. Oxygen should be administered via a low- to medium-concentration device. An intravenous should be initiated and run at TKVO. An ACP may administer analgesics if within local protocol.

En route to the hospital, the patient complains of more difficulty breathing and greater pain in the affected area. You assess her respiratory effort and observe that it is shallow as if there is guarding, but there is still equal air entry bilaterally. You observe paradoxical movement of the affected left side of the chest.

Treatment Continued

Based on your findings, the patient's affected ribs should be stabilized with a small towel or large pressure dressing. This dressing should be taped in place over the fractured segment so as not to impede breathing and to provide comfort. Constant re-evaluation of the patient's respiratory status and vital signs should continue en route to the hospital.

Differential Diagnosis

- Flail chest.

Test Your Knowledge

1. What is a flail chest?
2. Why did the flail chest not present immediately?
3. Given that the chest is not functioning as a bellows, why is there paradoxical movement of the affected left side?
4. What is the classification of the patient's medication?
5. What ECG does the patient present with?
6. What other damage may the patient be susceptible to?
7. In a flail chest, why does lung compliance eventually fall, and why is more pressure required to inflate the lung?

CASE 9.2

You are called to a residence at 1441 Prince Street, Rustico, Prince Edward Island, on a late fall afternoon for a patient with chest pain. On arrival, you find a female patient, approximately 36 years old, sitting on her front steps holding her chest. The patient, Natalie, has tears in her eyes. She tells you that she was involved in a car accident two days earlier, was taken to the hospital, and later released. She said she was told she had a few broken ribs in the front of her chest. The pain was bad yesterday but appears worse today, and it seems to her to be a different type of chest pain.

Initial Assessment Findings & Chief Complaint

LOA	Conscious and alert.
A	Patent.
B	Shallow but regular.
C	Strong radial pulses.
Wet Check	Unremarkable.
CC	Chest pain.

History

S	Complaining of substernal pressure.
A	None.
M	Toradol, Tylenol #2.
P	Healthy.
L	Lunch.
E	The patient was in a car accident two days earlier and suffered fractured ribs. She now complains of a new onset of substernal pain. The patient tells you that the pain is unbearable and nothing relieves it. She has taken a Toradol and Tylenol 2 without relief.

Assessment

H/N	No JVD, trachea midline, tenderness of neck on palpation.
Chest	Pain on palpation of anterior chest, equal air entry bilaterally.
ABD	Soft/non-tender.
Back	Unremarkable.
Pelvis	Stable.
Ext	Equal strength and mobility in all extremities.

Vitals

BP	126/78
P	70, regular
RR	18 shallow
Pupils	PERL 3+ mm
GCS	4+5+6=15
BS	n/a
Pulse oximetry	99%
Skin	Warm, dry

Pain Assessment

O	Gradually
P	While at rest
Q	Constant ache
R	Chest
S	8/10
T	Throughout the morning

Cardiac Monitor

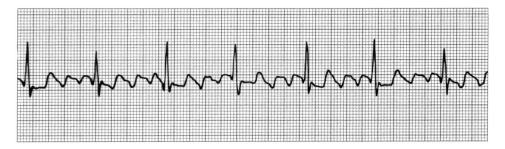

Figure 9.2

Initial Treatment Post Assessment

The patient should be assessed and a complete set of vitals obtained, including SPO2 and ECG interpretation. Oxygen should be administered via a high concentration mask and an intravenous should be secured and initiated at TKVO. The patient should then be placed in a position of comfort and transported to the nearest hospital. En route, an assessment and description of the chest pain should be obtained to rule out ischemia.

There is no change in the patient's condition or pain complaints en route to the hospital.

Differential Diagnosis

- Pulmonary contusion.

Test Your Knowledge

1. The complaint of chest pain that Natalie is presenting with is consistent with cardiac ischemia. How does one differentiate and treat this condition?
2. Should you concern yourself with c-spine precautions if the patient was seen in the ER two days earlier?
3. What better describes a blunt cardiac injury (BCI)-myocardial contusion?
4. What are the signs and symptoms of a BCI-myocardial contusion?
5. What classifications are the patient's medications?
6. What ECG is the patient presenting with?
7. Differentiate between a myocardial contusion and a commotio cordis.

Answers

Case 9.1

1. *What is a flail chest?*

   A flail chest occurs when three or more adjacent ribs are fractured in two or more places.

2. *Why did the flail chest not present immediately?*

   The flail chest did not present immediately as intercostal muscles spasmed and provided a natural splinting. As time progressed, the intercostal muscles suffered more injury, or fatigue set in, and the paradoxical movement became more evident. The administration of analgesics may also have caused the intercostal muscles to relax, contributing to a more noticeable finding.

3. *Given that the chest is not functioning as a bellows, why is there paradoxical movement of the affected left side?*

   The injury produces a movement that interferes with the continuation of the chest wall. The chest wall thus moves in the opposite direction from normal chest wall movement. The movement further reduces the air expelled by each breath and displaces the mediastinum toward and away from the injured site. As a result, the patient uses more energy to move less air.

4. *What is the classification of the patient's medication?*

   glyburide (Diabeta)   – Oral hypoglycemic

5. *What ECG does the patient present with?*

   The patient is presenting with a normal sinus rhythm.

6. *What other damage may the patient be susceptible to if not treated?*

   The patient's flail segment movement may damage surrounding tissue. As the patient breathes, the bone fracture sites move against one another, causing muscle and soft-tissue damage. Since a flail chest injury takes a substantial force, several underlying internal injuries often result.

7. *In a flail chest, why does lung compliance eventually fall, and why is more pressure required to inflate the lung?*

   Lung compliance eventually falls and more pressure is required to inflate the lung due to air moving into the area of the pulmonary contusion caused by the fractures.

Case 9.2

1. ***The complaint of chest pain that Natalie is presenting with is consistent with cardiac ischemia. How does one differentiate and treat this condition?***

   The patient may be complaining of chest or retrosternal chest pain that is very much like that of myocardial infarction. Relevant incident history should include significant chest trauma, particularly to the anterior chest. If there is any doubt and the patient is at high risk for cardiac ischemia, you should consider treating her as a cardiac patient.

2. ***Should you concern yourself with c-spine precautions if the patient was seen in the ER two days earlier?***

   The patient was taken to the hospital ER as an accident victim. In the ER, common procedures include ruling out c-spine injuries. C-spine precautions on this call should not be a concern.

3. ***What better describes a blunt cardiac injury (BCI)-myocardial contusion?***

   A myocardial contusion is a frequent result of chest trauma. Cardiac contusion is similar to contusion in any other muscle tissue: it results in muscle fibre tears and damage, hemorrhage, and edema. Cardiac contusion may result in a reduction in the strength and conductivity of the heart.

4. ***What are the signs and symptoms of a BCI-myocardial contusion?***

   Signs and symptoms of a myocardial contusion include:
   - Blunt injury to chest
   - Bruising of the wall of the chest
   - Rapid irregular heartbeat
   - Nagging pain in the chest not relieved with rest

5. ***What classifications are the patient's medications?***

   Toradol (ketorolac) — NSAID
   Tylenol 2 (acetaminophen with 15 mg codeine) — Narcotic analgesic

6. ***What ECG is the patient presenting with?***

   The patient is presenting with an atrial flutter.

7. ***Differentiate between a myocardial contusion and a commotio cordis.***

   Commotio cordis is the mechanical stimulation of the heart in the absence of structural damage, while myocardial contusion involves tissue damage. Commotio cordis is usually a sudden disturbance of the heart's rhythm and is observed more commonly in sports or as a result of non-penetrating impact. The impact is transmitted to the heart muscles and may in turn cause an arrhythmia or an ectopic beat. A myocardial contusion involves actual bruising of the heart.

Chapter 10
Abdominal Trauma

Injuries to the abdomen, whether blunt or penetrating, can cause damage to internal organs as well as possible hypovolemia. Because of the multitude of organs in this confined space, signs and symptoms of abdominal injuries may be limited or vague. The mechanism and quadrant of injury are therefore key components in the assessment of a patient. As the abdomen is an enclosed space, internal bleeding can occur without paramedics being able to provide care for it. The early recognizable signs and symptoms of shock should indicate any need for surgical intervention. Specific classifications of patients, such as pediatric or expectant mothers, are at an increased risk of life-threatening injuries.

CASE 10.1

You are dispatched at 02:15hrs to outside 23 Water Street, Harbour Grace, Newfoundland, for a possible stabbing. As you pull up to the curb, you observe a male in his forties holding his abdomen. His shirt is covered with blood. The police arrive at the same time and secure the scene as you approach. No weapon has been found. The patient tells you that a young punk tried to take his wallet and in the ensuing scuffle the patient saw a knife come out. The next thing he knew, he was cut and bleeding. The assailant ran away after not being able to get the patient's wallet.

Initial Assessment Findings & Chief Complaint

LOA	Conscious and alert.
A	Patent.
B	Regular and full volume.
C	Strong radial pulses.
Wet Check	The front of the patient's shirt is soaked with blood and there is a cut mark laterally across the lower front quadrant.
CC	Stabbing.

History

S	Laceration of the abdomen.
A	None.
M	Lipitor, Tylenol, Effexor, Imovane.
P	High cholesterol.
L	Supper.
E	Attacked by a stranger trying to take his wallet. In the process, the patient was cut across the abdomen with a knife.

Assessment

H/N	No JVD, trachea midline, no trauma noted.
Chest	Symmetrical, unremarkable with equal air entry and no adventitious sounds.
ABD	There is a laceration of approximately 15 cm across the abdomen and abdominal contents protruding. Bleeding at the site has subsided.
Back	Unremarkable.
Pelvis	Stable.
Ext	Blood on the hands but no trauma noted, with the exception of minor abrasions on the right knuckles. Lower extremities are unremarkable.

Vitals

BP	118/88
P	100 strong and irregular
RR	16 full volume
Pupils	PERL 3+ mm
GCS	4+5+6=15
BS	n/a
Pulse oximetry	98%
Skin	Warm, dry

Pain Assessment

O	n/a
P	n/a
Q	n/a
R	n/a
S	n/a
T	n/a

Cardiac Monitor

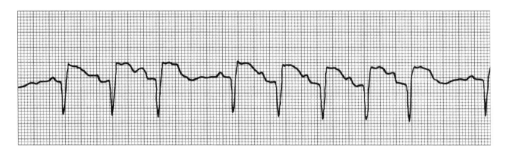

Figure 10.1

Initial Treatment Post Assessment

The patient should be moved to a stretcher and thoroughly assessed for additional injuries or stab wounds. A complete set of vitals and ECG interpretation should be obtained. Oxygen should be administered via a high concentration mask. The evisceration should be covered with sterile gauze dampened with sterile water or normal saline. The area should then be covered with an aluminum foil blanket to keep it wet and warm. The patient should be positioned so as to not apply additional pressure on the protruding part of his abdomen. An intravenous should be initiated en route to the hospital and run at TKVO.

En route, the patient complains of constant pain and is nauseated. There are no significant changes to his vital signs.

Treatment Continued

Reassessment of the patient should continue on the way to the hospital. There are no significant treatment differences for ACP or PCP care. Analgesics should not be administered.

Differential Diagnosis

- Evisceration of the abdomen.

Test Your Knowledge

1. With abdominal evisceration, what is likely to protrude?
2. Why is it not appropriate treatment to force the protrusion back into the abdominal cavity?
3. What ECG is the patient presenting with?
4. What are the classifications of the patient's medications?
5. What may be compromised as a result of the protrusion?
6. What other complications may develop with an abdominal evisceration?
7. If the police had not arrived and secured the scene, what would you have done as you arrived?

CASE 10.2

You are dispatched to the Welsh residence at 17:00hrs in Fogo, Newfoundland, for a six-year-old complaining of abdominal pain. On arrival, you meet Mrs. Welsh, who tells you that Henry, her son, has hurt his stomach. She reports that Henry was mountain biking and doing jumps when he landed hard on his handlebars. He fell to the ground, having apparently lost his wind, and lay there for a while feeling extremely sore. After about half an hour he began biking again and came home for lunch. After lunch, Henry complained of more pain and went to lie down. When his mother checked on him, his abdomen appeared swollen and Henry was in even more pain. As you approach Henry, you see that he is lying on the bed in a fetal position and appears pale.

Initial Assessment Findings & Chief Complaint

LOA	Conscious and alert.
A	Patent.
B	Shallow.
C	Strong radial pulse.
Wet Check	Unremarkable.
CC	Abdominal pain.

History

S	Abdominal pain from bike accident.
A	None.
M	Ritalin–SR.
P	ADHD.
L	Lunch.
E	Henry was biking and fell on his handlebars during a jump. He is now complaining of a swollen abdomen, pain, and nausea.

Assessment

H/N	Unremarkable.
Chest	Unremarkable, small abrasions on chest laterally along lower ribs.
ABD	Distended firm abdomen with an abrasion on the right upper quadrant (RUQ) and pain on palpation.
Back	Unremarkable.
Pelvis	Stable.
Ext	Equal strength and mobility in upper and lower extremities. Small abrasions and multiple older bruises on lower legs and knees.

Vitals

BP	90/60
P	150, regular
RR	18 shallow
Pupils	PERL 3+ mm
GCS	4+5+6=15
BS	n/a
Pulse oximetry	99%
Skin	Pale, dry

Pain Assessment

O	Increasing in severity
P	Fall on bike handlebars
Q	Constant pain, increased on movement
R	None
S	9/10
T	3 hours

Cardiac Monitor

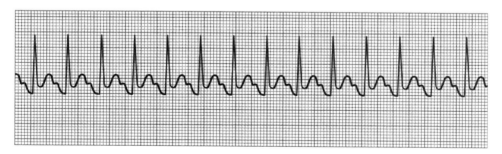

Figure 10.2

Initial Treatment Post Assessment

The patient should be assessed and a c-spine injury ruled out, if warranted. Oxygen should be administered via a high concentration mask. A complete set of vitals should be obtained, including SPO2. Cardiac monitoring should be initiated and continued en route to the clinic. The patient should be placed in a position of comfort in either a left lateral recumbent or knee-to-chest position. An intravenous should be initiated and run at TKVO. There are no specific treatment differences between ACP and PCP care.

En route, the patient lies motionless and continues to complain of pain. His vitals remain stable.

Differential Diagnosis

- Splenic injury (laceration or rupture).

Test Your Knowledge

1. What is significant about the patient's position when you arrive on scene?
2. What would be key to a successful interaction with a six-year-old?
3. Why are solid organs prone to fractures (ruptures) or contusions?
4. In pediatric patients, what provides protection to the spleen and diminishes with age?
5. Why are children more prone to splenic injuries than adults?
6. What is the classification of the patient's medication?
7. What ECG is the patient presenting with?
8. What is a typical compensatory response for a child with hypovolemia?

Answers

Case 10.1

1. *With an abdominal evisceration, what is likely to protrude?*

    With an abdominal evisceration, either or both the omentum and the small bowel are most likely to protrude.

2. *Why is it not appropriate treatment to force the protrusion back into the abdominal cavity?*

    It is not appropriate treatment to reinsert the protrusion into the abdominal cavity because doing so may introduce bacteria and other particles into the peritoneal space.

3. *What ECG is the patient presenting with?*

    The patient is presenting in a second-degree AV block, type 1.

4. *What are the classifications of the patient's medications?*

    | **Lipitor** (atorvastatin) | – Lipid metabolism regulator |
    | **Tylenol** (acetaminophen) | – Analgesic |
    | **Effexor** (venlafaxine hydrochloride) | – Antidepressant |
    | **Imovane** (zopiclone) | – Hypnotic |

5. *What may be compromised as a result of the protrusion?*

    Circulation may be compromised as the protruding part may have been tamponaded. Drying of the intra-abdominal tissue may also occur.

6. *What other complications may develop with an abdominal evisceration?*

    With an eviscerated abdomen, the patient risks the additional danger of peritonitis that might result from the contents of the bowel being cut or torn and leaking into the abdominal cavity.

7. *If the police had not arrived and secured the scene, what would you have done as you arrived?*

    Scene security and personal safety are the most important aspects of the daily routine of a paramedic. Upon arriving and observing the man on the sidewalk, the paramedics should have stayed in their vehicle until police arrived. Conversations with the man could have been carried out through a partially opened window. Given that the scene was unsecured, the appropriate course of action would have been to stay a short distance away and wait until it had been secured by police.

Case 10.2

1. ***What is significant about the patient's position when you arrive on scene?***

   The patient is lying motionless in a position of comfort. He is lying in a fetal position, which decreases the amount of pressure in the abdomen.

2. ***What would be key to a successful interaction with a six-year-old?***

   Keys to a successful interaction include involving the child in the assessment, respecting his or her modesty, and allowing the child to make treatment choices when possible.

3. ***Why are solid organs prone to fractures (ruptures) or contusions?***

   Solid organs are more prone to contusions or fractures because they are dense and not held together as strongly as muscular organs.

4. ***In pediatric patients, what provides protection to the spleen and diminishes with age?***

   Pediatric patients have a thicker capsule surrounding the solid organs, which minimizes the amount of bleeding in a blunt injury. If the capsule is penetrated, however, there will be no benefit from this extra thickness.

5. ***Why are children more prone to splenic injuries than adults?***

   The most common form of abdominal pediatric injury is blunt trauma. Liver and spleen injuries are more common in children compared to adults because these organs are relatively larger in children and not well-protected by the high, broad, costal arch of a child's ribs.

6. ***What is the classification of the patient's medication?***

   Ritalin-SR (methylphenidate)   – Stimulant

7. ***What ECG is the patient presenting with?***

   The patient is presenting with a sinus tachycardia.

8. ***What is a typical compensatory response for a child with hypovolemia?***

   The typical compensatory response for a child in hypovolemia is tachycardia.

Division 2 Medical Emergencies

Chapter 11
Pulmonary Emergencies

Respiratory distress can arise from a number of causes, including foreign substance inhalation, foreign body obstruction, anxiety and fear, and pain. Other pathologies include asthma, COPD, pulmonary edema, pulmonary embolism, and anaphylaxis. However, not all dyspnea stems from respiratory ailments. By keeping an open and investigative mind, paramedics can see past the visual presentation of dyspnea. Looking deeper into the possible pathology, a working assessment and differential diagnosis can be reached.

A general visual assessment of a patient upon arrival on scene may aid in understanding the cause of dyspnea. One of the most important pieces of information to obtain from a patient is the length of time he or she has had difficulty breathing. This information does not exclude other aspects of their history, but helps paint a clearer picture for the paramedic.

CASE 11.1

You are dispatched at 16:45hrs to a private residence at 22 Santa Monica Street, Sudbury, Ontario, for a 22-year-old female who is having difficulty breathing. Your response time is approximately five to seven minutes due to the traffic at this time of day. On arrival, you find the patient in her living room in a tripod position, attempting to breathe. A friend at the scene tells you that the patient has had increased breathing difficulties for four days and went to see a doctor at a walk-in clinic earlier that day. The patient was given a prescription for Becloforte and has taken two puffs.

Initial Assessment Findings & Chief Complaint

LOA	Patient is confused as to time.
A	Airway appears patent.
B	RR 20 shallow.
C	Radial pulses present at 126 bpm.
Wet Check	Unremarkable.
CC	Patient says she "can't catch her breath."

History

S	Distressed breathing over a period of four days.
A	None known by the patient.
M	salbutamol, glyburide, fluticasone. Becloforte today.
P	Diabetes, asthma.
L	Lunch.
E	Sitting relaxing throughout the day after returning from the doctor's office.

Assessment

H/N	No JVD, trachea midline, supraclavicular indrawing.
Chest	No A/E at the bases, and decreased A/E at the apexes with expiratory wheezing present.
ABD	Soft/non-tender, ABD muscle usage for breathing.
Back	Normal.
Pelvis	Normal.
Ext	Good ROM, capillary refill delayed, mottling present in lower extremities.

Vitals

BP	138/84
P	150 regular
RR	20 shallow
Pupils	3+ mm
GCS	4+4+6=14
BS	4.4 mmol/l
Pulse oximetry	88%
Skin	diaphoretic

Pain Assessment

O	n/a
P	n/a
Q	n/a
R	n/a
S	n/a
T	n/a

Cardiac Monitor

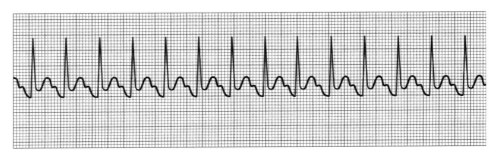

Figure 11.1

Initial Treatment Post Assessment

During assessment, the patient should be given 100% oxygen. After a complete history and vitals are obtained, including pulse oximetry and ECG interpretation, salbutamol 5.0 mg should be administered via a nebulizer or metered dose inhaler (MDI). Dosages vary, but a patient can receive up to 900 μg (one puff = 100 μg of salbutamol). The patient should be placed in a position that maximizes air exchange and transported as soon as possible.

En route to the hospital, the patient's breathing worsens, with decreased A/E and evidence of bronchoconstriction with decreased expiratory wheezing and lethargy. The patient's vitals remain unchanged with the exception of her respiratory rate, which is now 11 and shallow. The patient's skin is still mottled and peripheral cyanosis is now present. She is becoming extremely agitated and fearful.

Treatment Continued

The paramedic might anticipate that the patient may require ventilation. Subcutaneous epinephrine may be administered (0.3–0.5 mg) as per local protocol. Administration of oxygen should be continued and additional epinephrine may be administered. If at any time the patient cannot control her airway or becomes unconscious, an oropharyngeal airway, nasopharyngeal airway, laryngeal mask, or combitube should be utilized. An Advanced Care Paramedic should intubate to secure the patient's airway. Salbutamol may then be administered via ETT.

Differential Diagnosis

- Asthma.

Test Your Knowledge

1. What is significant about the patient's position when you arrive on scene?
2. What are the classifications of the patient's medications?
3. What is significant about the new medication prescribed by the physician at the clinic?
4. The treatment includes salbutamol administered via a nebulizer. What are the possible adverse reactions to this medication?
5. What are the typical signs and symptoms that asthmatics present with?
6. What is the cause of the decreased breathing sounds in the apexes and, eventually, throughout (silent chest)?
7. Is your patient's condition acute or chronic? How do you know?
8. What ECG is the patient presenting with?

CASE 11.2

You are dispatched at 20:00hrs to the YMCA in Nanaimo, British Columbia, for a 25-year-old male who was playing basketball and now has pain in his chest and difficulty breathing. You arrive at the scene approximately seven minutes after receiving the call. Upon arrival, you notice a tall man sitting on a bench, clutching the right side of his chest and breathing rapidly. He introduces himself as Scott Thompson. He tells you it hurts more when he breathes deeply. He is pale and diaphoretic, and reports that he had been playing ball for approximately 30 minutes before the pain came on.

Initial Assessment Findings & Chief Complaint

LOA	Patient is alert and oriented x3.
A	Airway is patent.
B	RR 24 shallow.
C	Radial pulse present at 116 bpm.
Wet Check	Unremarkable.
CC	Pain in chest, difficulty breathing.

History

S	Sudden, sharp pain in right side of chest and difficulty catching his breath.
A	None.
M	None.
P	None.
L	Supper three hours earlier.
E	Playing a game of basketball.

Assessment

H/N	No JVD, trachea is midline.
Chest	Decreased breath sounds on right side of chest, accessory muscle usage.
ABD	Soft/non-tender, abdominal muscle usage to breathe.
Back	Normal.
Pelvis	Normal.
Ext	Capillary refill is normal.

Vitals

BP	110/70
P	150 strong/regular
RR	24 shallow/laboured
Pupils	3+ mm
GCS	4+5+6=15
BS	4.1 mmol/l
Pulse oximetry	90%
Skin	Pale/diaphoretic

Pain Assessment

O	Right side of chest
P	Playing basketball
Q	Sharp, worse on inspiration
R	Doesn't radiate
S	6/10
T	15 minutes

Cardiac Monitor

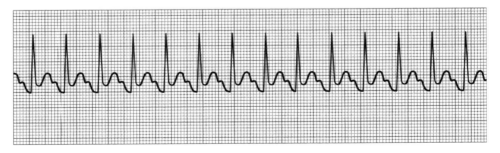

Figure 11.2

Initial Treatment Post Assessment

During assessment, the patient should be placed on high concentration oxygen via a non-breather mask. After a complete history and vitals are obtained, the patient should be positioned to maximize air exchange and transported as soon as possible. An intravenous should be secured and infused TKVO.

En route to the hospital, the patient's breathing becomes more laboured. Breath sounds on the right side of his chest are now shallower. The patient is becoming more agitated and confused. His pulse is now 120 and his BP is 120/70. His respiratory rate is 12. He is also more diaphoretic and is becoming cyanotic.

Treatment Continued

Supportive care ECG monitoring should continue en route. ACPs and PCPs should carry out reassessment of the trachea and auscultation of the lung fields. SPO2 and other vitals should also be monitored during transport.

Differential Diagnosis

- Pneumothorax (spontaneous).

Test Your Knowledge

1. The patient is sitting upright on a bench when you arrive. Why?
2. The patient has no previous medical history. What could have caused his pneumothorax?
3. What other problems might present with similar signs and symptoms?
4. What are the risk factors for developing spontaneous pneumothorax?
5. What are the typical signs and symptoms of pneumothorax?
6. What cardiac rhythm is the patient presenting in?

CASE 11.3

You are dispatched priority 4 at 14:30hrs to a residence at 571 Bloom Street, Flin Flon, Manitoba, for a 65-year-old male complaining of shortness of breath. Upon arrival at the scene, you observe the patient sitting upright on a couch in a tripod position. You notice the patient is on home oxygen and seems to be having trouble catching his breath. The patient explains that he has been a pack-a-day smoker for close to 20 years and has been having trouble breathing since he got up at 08:30hrs this morning. The patient is on home oxygen via nasal cannula at 2 lpm.

Initial Assessment Findings & Chief Complaint

LOA	Patient is confused as to time and date.
A	Airway is patent.
B	RR 24 shallow, laboured with accessory muscle usage.
C	Radial and carotid present at a rate of 150 bpm, irregular.
Wet Check	Unremarkable.
CC	Patient cannot catch his breath.

History

S	Increased difficulty breathing since waking.
A	No known allergies.
M	salbutamol, Beconase.
P	Asthma, emphysema.
L	Dinner the previous night.
E	Patient woke up in bed with difficulty breathing.

Assessment

H/N	No JVD, trachea is midline, supraclavicular indrawing, purse-lipped breathing.
Chest	Patient has decreased breathing sounds throughout and expiratory wheezing in apexes, and appears barrel-chested.
ABD	Soft/non-tender with abdominal muscle usage to breathe.
Back	Unremarkable.
Pelvis	Unremarkable.
Ext	Peripheral cyanosis, delayed capillary refill.

Vitals

Pain Assessment

BP	164/100	O	N/A
P	150, irregular	P	N/A
RR	24 shallow, laboured	Q	N/A
Pupils	PERL 3+ mm	R	N/A
GCS	4+4+6=14	S	N/A
BS	4.8 mmol/l	T	N/A
Pulse oximetry	89%		
Skin	Cool, dry		

Cardiac Monitor

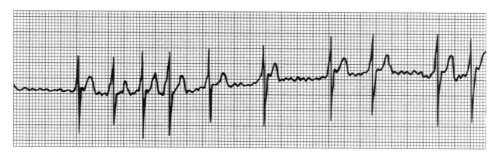

Figure 11.3

Initial Treatment Post Assessment

The patient should be put on high flow oxygen via a nonrebreather at 12 lpm and transported in an upright position in order to aid his breathing. A pulse oximeter should be utilized to continually monitor the patient's oxygen saturation, and a cardiac monitor should be applied. ACP and PCP treatment may include administering medications such as metaproterenol and salbutamol and initiating an intravenous running at TKVO. A blood glucometry should also be obtained.

En route to the hospital, the patient's breathing begins to improve slightly, and his respiratory rate decreases to 18. His heart rate also slows to 110, and his blood pressure drops down to 140/86. The patient's level of awareness improves and he is now at a GCS of 15. Peripheral cyanosis is no longer present and all other vitals remain the same.

Treatment Continued

Administration of bronchodilators should continue en route until breathing is eased. Oxygen administration via nasal cannula at 24–28% can be continued.

Differential Diagnosis

- Emphysema.

Test Your Knowledge

1. What are the typical signs and symptoms of emphysema?
2. Is your patient's condition acute or chronic? How do you know?
3. What cardiac rhythm is the patient presenting in?
4. A treatment of an acute exacerbation of emphysema may include salbutamol. What is the mechanism of action of this drug when administered to a patient with emphysema?

5. Would a blood glucometry be beneficial for this patient during the primary assessment or during a post treatment assessment?
6. What is the classification of the other medication the patient is taking?

CASE 11.4

You are dispatched at 12:30hrs to a local music museum in Spring Hill, Nova Scotia, for an 80-year-old female who has had a syncopal episode and now has difficulty breathing. Your response time is approximately 10 minutes because of traffic. On arrival, the patient is sitting in an upright position, surrounded by two friends who are comforting her as she tries to breathe. The patient's friends tell you that Marie seemed fine until suddenly her legs gave out and she collapsed. They caught her before she hit the floor. When Marie awoke, she was having difficulty breathing and was grabbing her chest because of intense pain. Her friends tell you that they are visiting from England and arrived yesterday on a long flight.

Initial Assessment Findings & Chief Complaint

LOA	Patient is confused as to date and day of the week.
A	Airway is patent.
B	RR 24 shallow and laboured.
C	Radial and carotid are present although weak, thready and irregular.
Wet Check	Unremarkable.
CC	Laboured breathing and temporary loss of consciousness (syncope).

History

S	Feeling tired today, sore lower leg, warm to touch, and shortness of breath.
A	None.
M	Lipitor, Aldactazide, Tylenol.
P	Kidney disease, hypertension, high cholesterol, and hip surgery five weeks prior.
L	Lunch.
E	Collapsed while at the music museum.

Assessment

H/N	No JVD, trachea is midline.
Chest	Equal air entry, shallow, laboured breaths.
ABD	Soft/non-tender.
Back	Unremarkable.
Pelvis	Unremarkable.
Ext	Good motor, swollen lower left leg.

Vitals

BP	146/92
P	150, irregular
RR	24 shallow, laboured
Pupils	PERL 3+ mm
GCS	4+4+5=13
BS	5.2 mmol/l
Pulse oximetry	93%
Skin	Pale, diaphoretic

Pain Assessment

O	Sudden
P	Nothing
Q	Sharp
R	None
S	9/10
T	20 minutes

Cardiac Monitor

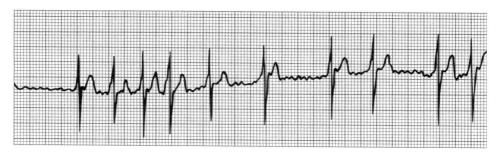

Figure 11.4

Initial Treatment Post Assessment

During primary assessment, the patient should be administered oxygen via a high concentration mask. A complete set of vitals should be obtained, including a cardiac monitor and blood glucometry. The patient should be moved to a stretcher, placed in the most comfortable position, and promptly transported to hospital. Ongoing assessment of the patient should continue en route. An intravenous should be initiated and infused at TKVO.

En route, the patient's breathing begins to deteriorate and she complains of acute sharp pain in her left chest. Her respiratory rate increases to 28 and shallow, and she eventually stops breathing. Her heart rate slows to a modest 30, and she has no palpable blood pressure.

Cardiac Monitor

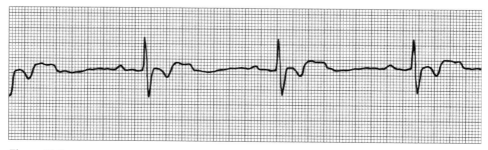

Figure 11.5

Treatment Continued

The patient requires ventilation as soon as possible with a BVM post airway adjunct. The ACP should intubate to secure the patient's airway (ETT 7.0, 21–22 cm at the teeth) and ventilate with the BVM to assess compliance. Atropine (0.5–1.0 mg), although generally contraindicated in this rhythm, may be beneficial. External pacing may also be a treatment option. Because of the patient's now hypotensive state, an IV bolus should be initiated. Continued aggressive oxygenation and monitoring is required throughout transport. Ongoing circulation assessment is required as there is potential for PEA.

Differential Diagnosis

- Pulmonary embolism.

Test Your Knowledge

1. What is significant about the patient's position when you arrive at the scene?
2. What classifications are the patient's medications?
3. Why is a pulmonary embolism hard to detect in a pre-hospital setting?
4. What signs and symptoms are most important in helping to determine a pulmonary embolism?
5. What cardiac rhythm is the patient presenting in?
6. What is the most important role for a paramedic if a pulmonary embolism is suspected?

CASE 11.5

You are dispatched at 14:30hrs on a Sunday afternoon to Monteith Correctional Facility in Ontario for a 51-year-old male having difficulty breathing. Your response time to the call is approximately six minutes. On arrival, the patient, Bob, is found sitting on his bed in his cell with his hands on his knees and elbows straight. He has been feeling generally unwell and has had a fever and severe cough for the past few days.

Initial Assessment Findings & Chief Complaint

LOA	Altered, confused as to time and date.
A	Patent.
B	Shallow and laboured at 24.
C	Weak and irregular radial pulse.
Wet Check	Unremarkable.
CC	Difficulty breathing with productive cough.

History

S	The patient has been complaining of feeling hot, sweaty, and generally unwell for the past few days. The previous day he began coughing up yellow phlegm. He has the chills and has had difficulty breathing.
A	NKA.
M	flecainide, verapamil.
P	Cardiac dysrhythmias.
L	Lunch.
E	Bob worked out in the fields in the rain for several days the previous week as part of his work assignment. He was allowed to stay inside today and not report to his work detail. When he started complaining of increased difficulty breathing, the warden called 911.

Assessment

H/N	No head trauma, trachea midline, no JVD.
Chest	Decreased air entry to bases with expiratory wheezing, indrawing, and accessory muscle usage.
ABD	Soft/non-tender, accessory muscle usage.
Back	Unremarkable.
Pelvis	Unremarkable.
Ext	Cool to touch.

Vitals

BP	108/68
P	130, irregular
RR	24
Pupils	PERL 4+ mm
GCS	4+4+6=14
BS	6.2 mmol/l
Pulse oximetry	84%
Skin	Febrile, with cool extremities

Pain Assessment

O	None
P	n/a
Q	n/a
R	n/a
S	n/a
T	n/a

Cardiac Monitor

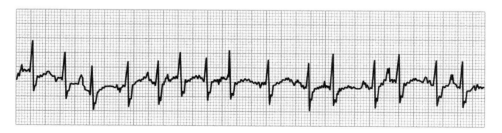

Figure 11.6

Initial Treatment Post Assessment

After an initial assessment, the patient should be administered oxygen via a high concentration mask. Cardiac monitoring and a blood glucometry should be completed. Because of his acute respiratory difficulty, the patient should be given a bronchodilator such as 900 μg salbutamol via MDI. Nebulized salbutamol should be avoided at this time. The patient should be transported in a position of comfort, and an intravenous should be initiated en route to the hospital and run at TKVO. Personal protective equipment (PPE) should be utilized throughout this call.

The patient's oxygen saturation has improved to 91%. He is still coughing up yellow phlegm and tells you he feels tired.

Treatment Continued

The patient needs to be continually monitored en route and additional salbutamol may be administered if his respiratory difficulties persist.

Differential Diagnosis

- Pneumonia of unknown etiology.

Test Your Knowledge

1. What is significant about the patient's position when you arrive on scene?
2. What classifications are the patient's medications?
3. What are the causes of pneumonia?
4. What are the typical symptoms of pneumonia?
5. What are the diagnostic methods for pneumonia?
6. What is the normal treatment regimen for bacterial pneumonia?
7. What is the patient's ECG interpretation?
8. Why should salbutamol not be administered by nebulizer in the treatment of this patient?

Answers

Case 11.1

1. *What is significant about the patient's position when you arrive on scene?*
   The patient is presenting in the tripod position when paramedics arrive, which maximizes the space within the chest and is the most adventitious for a respiratory distressed patient. By utilizing this position, the patient is attempting to maximize the effect of each breath.

2. *What are the classifications of the patient's medications?*

   salbutamol (Ventolin) — Beta-2 agonist
   fluticasone (Flovent) — Inhaled steroid
   Becloforte (beclomethasone dipropionate) — Corticosteroid
   glyburide (Diabeta) — Oral hypoglycemic

3. *What is significant about the new medication prescribed by the physician at the clinic?*

   A Becloforte inhaler (beclomethasone dipropionatey) is used for prophylactic management in asthma. Daily use as directed may prevent the frequency and severity of asthma attacks.

4. *The treatment included salbutamol administration via a nebulizer. What are the possible adverse reactions to this medication?*

   Adverse reactions to salbutamol include trembling, nervousness, flushing, and dysrhythmias due to the drug's stimulation of the beta-2 receptors in smooth muscle.

5. *What are the typical signs and symptoms that asthmatics present with?*

   The typical signs and symptoms presenting in asthmatics are
   Pulsus paradoxus: An exaggerated fall in systolic blood pressure during inspiration; may occur during acute asthma exacerbation.
   Wheezing: End-expiratory wheezing or a prolonged expiratory phase is most common, although inspiratory wheezing can be heard.
   Diminished breath sounds and chest hyperinflation: May be observed during acute exacerbations.

6. *What is the cause of the decreased breathing sounds in the apexes and, eventually, throughout (silent chest)?*

   The silent chest results from severe bronchoconstriction in the patient's airways.

7. *Is your patient's condition acute or chronic? How do you know?*

   The patient's condition is currently acute. A condition such as asthma is a chronic disease which can usually be controlled by prophylactic medications. This patient is hypoxic due to severe bronchoconstriction and needs urgent intervention.

8. *What ECG is the patient presenting with?*

   The patient is presenting with a sinus tachycardia.

Case 11.2

1. *The patient is sitting upright on a bench when you arrive. Why?*

   The patient is presenting in a sitting position, which is a position of comfort. He is not as active as he was, and he is concentrating on his chest discomfort.

2. *The patient has no previous medical history. What could have caused his pneumothorax?*

   The most common cause of a spontaneous pneumothorax is the rupture of air- or fluid-filled blisters on the surface of the lungs. This creates an opening into the pleural space, allowing air to enter.

3. *What other problems might present with similar signs and symptoms?*

   Decreased air entry can have many causes. Pulmonary embolism and aspiration are likely. Most other respiratory problems also present with tachypnea and tachycardia.

4. *What are the risk factors for developing spontaneous pneumothorax?*

   Risk factors for developing pneumothorax include:
   Tall, thin, and male
   History of smoking
   Family history
   Other respiratory illnesses

5. **What are the typical signs and symptoms of pneumothorax?**

   Typical signs and symptoms of pneumothorax may include:
   - Dyspnea
   - Sharp pain that is usually worse on inspiration or coughing
   - Decreased lung sounds on affected side
   - Tachycardia
   - Tachypnea
   - Anxiety

6. **What cardiac rhythm is the patient presenting in?**

   The patient is presenting in a sinus tachycardia.

Case 11.3

1. **What are the typical signs and symptoms of emphysema?**

   Patients presenting with emphysema present certain characteristic signs and symptoms, with an acute episode of worsening dyspnea that began while they were at rest. The patient is often sitting upright and leaning forward and has noticeable accessory muscle usage. They may present with the following signs and symptoms:
   - Tachycardia
   - Diaphoresis
   - Confusion
   - Irritability
   - Dyspnea
   - Wheezing on expiration or inspiration
   - Crackles can also be found in the lung fields
   - May appear thin and barrel-chested

2. **Is your patient's condition acute or chronic? How do you know?**

   The patient's underlying pathology of having emphysema is chronic. Emphysema is a disease that develops and worsens over time.

3. **What ECG is the patient presenting in?**

   The patient is presenting in an atrial fibrillation.

4. **A treatment of an acute exacerbation of emphysema may include salbutamol. What is the mechanism of action of this drug when administered to a patient with emphysema?**

   Salbutamol is a sympathomimetic, which is selective for beta-2 adrenergic receptors. It relaxes the smooth muscle of the bronchial tree and peripheral vasculature by stimulating the adrenergic receptors of the sympathetic nervous system.

5. **Would a blood glucometry be beneficial for this patient during the primary assessment or during a post treatment assessment?**

   A blood glucometry should always be performed during the primary assessment of a patient presenting with an altered level of awareness. Glucose is a key factor in the metabolic activities of the body, and if glucose levels are altered, this change may trigger other presenting conditions. The decreased oxygen saturation and chief complaint leads to the conclusion that the confusion may be caused by hypoxia.

6. **What is the classification of the other medication the patient is taking?**

   Beconase (beclomethasone)   – Nasal corticosteroid

Case 11.4

1. What is significant about the patient's position when you arrive at the scene?

The patient is presenting in an upright position when paramedics arrive. This is the best possible position for most patients in respiratory distress, because it allows the air entry to function at maximum efficiency.

2. What classification are the patient's medications?

Lipitor (atorvastatin) — Treatment of hypercholesterolemia
Aldactazide (spironolactone/HCT) — Diuretic
Tylenol (acetaminophen) — Analgesic

3. Why is a pulmonary embolism hard to detect in a pre-hospital setting?

Pulmonary embolism may be difficult to diagnose in a pre-hospital setting because its symptoms may occur with or appear similar to other conditions, such as a heart attack, panic attack, or pneumonia.

4. What signs and symptoms are most important in helping to determine a pulmonary embolism?

The most important signs and symptoms are usually associated with current medical history, such as previous surgery (especially hip surgery). Specific signs and symptoms may include:
   Pain in lower leg(s)
   Shortness of breath that may occur suddenly
   Sudden sharp chest pain
   Coughing
   Tachycardia
   Diaphoresis
   Heart palpitations
   Syncope

5. What cardiac rhythm is the patient presenting in?

The patient is presenting in an atrial fibrillation and later, en route, in a second-degree AV block, type 2.

6. What is the most important role for a paramedic if a pulmonary embolism is suspected?

The most important role for a paramedic if a PE is suspected is one of support. You must keep the patient's airway well supported and monitor respirations and any other changes. PE patients can deteriorate quickly, so you must be thoroughly prepared. Rapid transport to a hospital is the best option.

Case 11.5

1. What is significant about the patient's position when you arrive on scene?

The patient is expanding his chest cavity by manipulating his postural stance, which increases the volume capacity of his thoracic cavity and decreases abdominal resistance.

2. What classifications are the patient's medications?

felcainide (Tambocor) — Antidysrhythmic
verapamil (Isoptin) — Calcium channel blocker

3. What are the causes of pneumonia?

There are extrinsic and intrinsic factors that can cause pneumonia, including bacterial, viral, and fungal causes. The most common bacterial cause is Streptococcus pneumoniae.

4. *What are the typical symptoms of pneumonia?*

   The typical signs and symptoms of pneumonia include:
   Typical common presentation or complaints
   Fever
   Shaking chills
   Cough with associated sputum (productive cough)
   Possible pleuritic pain with deep breath, because of coughing

5. *What are the diagnostic methods for pneumonia?*

   Pneumonia is clinically diagnosed using a chest X-ray. One field assessment that might help a paramedic in coming to a working diagnosis of pneumonia is auscultation of the chest revealing crackles, wheezing, or diminished breath sounds. The patient will also usually present with a fever.

6. *What is the normal treatment regimen for bacterial pneumonia?*

   Bacterial pneumonia is usually treated with broad spectrum antibiotics such as ampicillin or amoxicillin.

7. *What is the patient's ECG interpretation?*

   The patient is presenting with a multifocal atrial tachycardia.

8. *Why should salbutamol not be administered by nebulizer in the treatment of this patient?*

   The risk of airborne infection is greater with a nebulizer than with MDI (metred dose inhaler) administration. This particular patient has signs and symptoms of a respiratory infection and is febrile; therefore, an MDI should be used to deliver the appropriate medications. Paramedics treating this patient should utilize personal protective equipment (PPE) such as gloves, a mask, and a gown to avoid contamination or infection.

Chapter 12
Cardiology

Cardiovascular disease is the number one cause of death in North America. Because of our aging population, the incidence of cardiovascular disease is expected to continue growing. Public education about early warnings, signs and symptoms, and risk factor recognition has been proven to increase survival rates and prevent sudden death. Time is of the essence when managing a possible ischemic heart disease patient. For the paramedic, early recognition, assessment, and treatment methods including oxygenation, platelet inhibitor administration, 12-lead ECG interpretation, and the use of medications to decrease preload will all increase a patient's chances of survival or minimize ongoing damage to the heart.

CASE 12.1

At 04:30hrs on a cold January morning, you are dispatched to a nursing home at 10 Riverview Drive, Gambo, Newfoundland, for a patient with severe dyspnea. On arrival, you are greeted by a nurse's aide, who points you in the direction of the patient's room. She does not know much about the patient but says she will meet you shortly in the patient's room with her chart. As you enter the private room, you observe the patient's name, Margaret Cole, on the door. Mrs. Cole appears to be in her mid-70s, and is lying in bed with three pillows under her head. The head of the bed appears to be sitting on two blocks of wood. She seems quite winded and grey. You are about 30 minutes from a hospital.

Initial Assessment Findings & Chief Complaint

LOA	Conscious, alert.
A	Appears patent.
B	Shallow, with audible crackles present.
C	Strong, irregular radial pulse.
Wet Check	Patient is wearing incontinence briefs.
CC	Respiratory distress.

History

S	Complaining of severe shortness of breath, denies chest pain.
A	Codeine, penicillin, walnuts, peanuts, fabric softener.
M	Altace, Norvasc, digoxin, Zestoretic, NTG, Zoloft, flurbiprofen, Diamox.
P	Glaucoma, hypertension, CHF. Similar occurrence of nocturnal dyspnea (CHF) two months earlier and was hospitalized and treated with BPAP.
L	Supper at 18:00hrs last night.
E	The patient awoke with extreme shortness of breath and called the nurse. The nurse administered oxygen via a non-rebreather mask until the tank ran dry moments before your arrival.

Assessment

H/N	JVD present, trachea midline.
Chest	Symmetrical with accessory muscle usage and coarse crackles from apex to bases bilaterally.
ABD	Soft/non-tender with an old midline surgical scar from the epigastric area distally to groin and around the umbilicus.
Back	Unremarkable, although mild mottling is present.
Pelvis	Stable.
Ext	Equal strength bilaterally in upper and lower extremities with pitting edema (class 4) in both ankles, progressing to mid-calves.

Vitals

BP	200/160
P	150 irregular
RR	28 shallow
Pupils	PERL 3+ mm
GCS	4+5+6=15
BS	n/a
Pulse oximetry	88%
Skin	Pale, grey, diaphoretic

Pain Assessment

O	n/a
P	n/a
Q	n/a
R	n/a
S	n/a
T	n/a

Cardiac Monitor

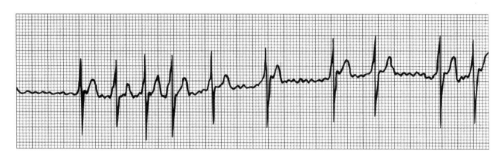

Figure 12.1

Initial Treatment Post Assessment

Because of the patient's severe dyspnea and colour, she should be administered oxygen via a high concentration mask, post SP02. After vitals have been obtained and a thorough assessment performed, the patient should be moved to a position that will improve respirations. An intravenous should be initiated and infused at TKVO. The patient's severe pulmonary edema should be treated with NTG 0.4–0.8 mg administered sublingually every five minutes. An ACP could administer a diuretic such as furosemide. The patient should be transported in a high fowler's position to a waiting ambulance. Because of the severely cold weather, the patient's face should be covered to prevent her from breathing cold air, which might lead to a cold-induced respiratory arrest.

En route to the hospital, there is no significant change in the patient's condition and her vitals remain the same.

Treatment Continued

The patient should continue to be treated with NTG and receive supplemental oxygen. If her respiratory status changes or she becomes lethargic, her respirations should be assisted with a bag-valve mask, providing positive pressure ventilations.

Differential Diagnosis

- Congestive heart failure.

Test Your Knowledge

1. What is significant about the patient's position when you arrive on scene?
2. What are the typical signs and symptoms of congestive heart failure?
3. The patient is taking several medications. What are their classifications?
4. Why do episodes of congestive heart failure occur so frequently in the early morning hours?
5. What cardiac rhythm is the patient presenting with?
6. How does the administration of NTG help this patient?
7. Why has diuretic therapy become "old school" in the treatment of CHF patients, although it may be beneficial in some instances?
8. Why should the patient not be positioned supine on your stretcher for transport to the emergency department?

CASE 12.2

You are dispatched at 21:00hrs to Pizza Delight, Saulnierville, for a patient who has fainted. It is just past the supper hour and the restaurant is starting to clear. You are greeted by a very anxious waiter who tells you that Mr. and Mrs. Thibeault were having supper when Stella Thibeault appeared to faint into her rappie pie. You see people standing around the patient's table. Stella is awake but appears confused and her skin looks pale and grey. As you approach, she asks why you are here. You explain that she fainted and she argues to the contrary. After a brief discussion, she allows you to assess her. She tells you that she has not been feeling well for the past hour, has difficulty breathing, and that her left hand hurts.

Initial Assessment Findings & Chief Complaint

LOA	Conscious, but appears confused.
A	Patent.
B	Shallow, slightly laboured at 24.
C	Weak, radial pulse.
Wet Check	Unremarkable.
CC	Weakness, syncope, difficulty breathing.

History

S	Patient complains of extreme weakness and has had difficulty breathing for the past 60 minutes.
A	Advil.
M	NTG patch, cardizem, paxil, Ativan, Xanax, glyburide, Prevacid, NTG, Tylenol.
P	Heart attack two years ago, angina, anxiety, diabetes, esophageal reflux, hip replacement three years ago.
L	Has eaten half of her supper.
E	Stella came to the restaurant feeling weak, began to eat, and had an onset of difficulty breathing. Her hand then became numb and tingly. She apparently fainted, and her lips turned blue for approximately 30 seconds.

Assessment

H/N	No JVD, trachea midline.
Chest	Equal air entry bilaterally although laboured breathing.
ABD	Soft/non-tender.
Back	Unremarkable.
Pelvis	Stable.
Ext	Equal strength and mobility.

Vitals

BP	80/60
P	50, regular
RR	24
Pupils	PERL 3+ mm
GCS	4+4+6=14
BS	6.2 mmol/l
Pulse oximetry	92%
Skin	Extremely pale and diaphoretic

Pain Assessment

O	n/a
P	n/a
Q	n/a
R	n/a
S	n/a
T	n/a

Cardiac Monitor

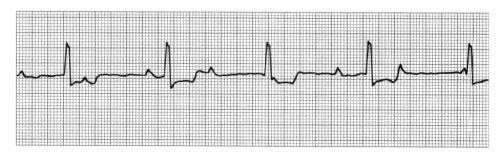

Figure 12.2

Initial Treatment Post Assessment

During primary assessment, the patient should receive oxygen via a non-rebreather mask. Cardiac monitoring and a blood glucometry should be completed. An intravenous should be established and a fluid bolus of 20 ml/kg initiated. An ACP should prepare the patient for transcutaneous pacing with sedation of minimal amounts of fentanyl or midazolam. The patient's blood pressure is below 100 systolic, so caution must be used when administering analgesics or sedatives. If pacing does not adequately increase her blood pressure, an infusion of Dopamine (5–10 µg/kg) can be established in addition to the fluid bolus. The patient should be transported in a position of comfort, and supine if possible.

En route to the hospital, the patient complains of difficulty breathing and hand pain, as well as 8 out of 10 chest pain. There is no change in the patient's ECG, but her blood pressure has increased to approximately 100 systolic.

Treatment continued

Treatment should continue and dopamine should be titrated to maintain a blood pressure of 100 systolic. Although her presentation is ischemic in nature, ASA should not be given because of her allergy to NSAIDs.

Differential Diagnosis

- AMI with cardiogenic shock.

Test Your Knowledge

1. Why is Stella argumentative when you arrive on scene?
2. What are the classifications of the patient's medications?
3. What is your interpretation of the patient's ECG?
4. What would be the best way to move the patient from her chair to a stretcher for transport?
5. What may have caused the patient to faint?
6. Could Stella be presenting with cardiac insufficiency or an AMI?
7. Why is Stella's blood pressure so low?

CASE 12.3

You are dispatched at 13:10hrs to 14 Main Street, Uranium City, Saskatchewan, for a 72-year-old male complaining of chest pain. En route, dispatch tells you that the male patient is in the upstairs apartment at the rear of the building. As you pull into the driveway, you see narrow, steep stairs leading to the apartment. You exit the vehicle and load your equipment. As you enter the unkempt apartment, you notice the patient, who is obese and weighs approximately 150 kg, sitting at a kitchen table. He is extremely diaphoretic and pale. The patient tells you his name is Don. He appears alert.

Initial Assessment Findings & Chief Complaint

LOA	Conscious, alert.
A	Patent.
B	Shallow at 16.
C	Strong radial pulse.
Wet Check	Unremarkable.
CC	Chest pain.

History

S	Patient complains of substernal pressure and sweating for approximately three hours, starting just after he had breakfast.
A	None.
M	Plendil, Lopressor, NTG, Glucophage, Dilantin, Naprosyn.
P	Hypertension, diabetes, arthritis, inguinal hernia repair five years prior.
L	Breakfast at 09:30hrs consisting of bacon, eggs, baked beans, and toast.
E	Approximately 30 minutes after eating, the patient became extremely diaphoretic and had an ache in his chest and neck. He took an antacid and thought it would be relieved. Half an hour later he vomited, and when the discomfort did not ease he called 911.

Assessment

H/N	No JVD, trachea midline.
Chest	Unremarkable, equal air entry with no adventitious sounds.
ABD	Soft/non-tender.
Back	Unremarkable.
Pelvis	Stable.
Ext	Equal strength/mobility in extremities.

Vitals

BP	132/90
P	170, regular
RR	16, shallow
Pupils	PERL 3+ mm
GCS	4+5+6=15
BS	n/a
Pulse oximetry	94%
Skin	Pale, diaphoretic

Pain Assessment

O	After eating breakfast
P	At rest
Q	Pressure, ache
R	Jaw
S	8/10
T	3 hours

Cardiac Monitor

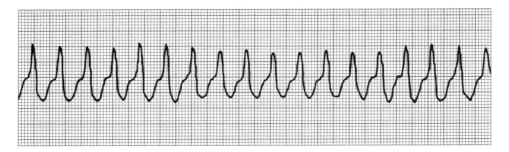

Figure 12.3

Initial Treatment Post Assessment

Post assessment, the patient should be given supplemental oxygen via a high concentration mask. Continual monitoring of vital signs should be performed, and an ECG interpretation should be completed. Since the patient does not have any allergies, ASA 160 mg should be administered by mouth. An intravenous should be initiated and run at TKVO. The patient should be placed in a comfortable position on a stretcher after being moved down the stairs with a stairchair or other extrication device. Additional resources may be required because of the patient's weight. Sublingual nitroglycerin should be administered every five minutes for ischemic chest pain. An ACP should administer morphine to the patient when he complains of ongoing pain. Rapid transport to an emergency facility should be carried out while monitoring vital signs and reassessing quality of ischemic pain.

En route, the patient vomits and becomes unconscious. You assess the patient and his vital signs are now presenting in the following rhythm.

Cardiac Monitor

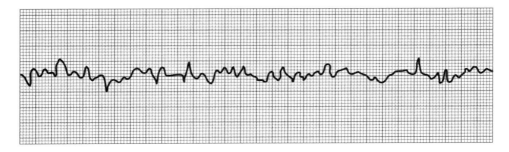

Figure 12.4

Treatment Continued

You should suction the remnants of the patient's breakfast to ensure patency of his airway. An airway adjunct such as an OPA or combitube can be inserted and CPR started while assessing ventilatory compliance. Defibrillator pads should be applied in the apex-sternum position and the patient should be defibrillated as soon as possible. A cardiac arrest protocol should be followed according to local policies. At the conclusion of CPR, the patient should be reanalyzed and defibrillated as required. An ACP should administer epinephrine, followed by an anti-arrhythmic such as lidocaine or amiodarone after the next session of CPR, post shock. Shock-drug-shock protocol should be followed. Endotrachial intubation and tube confirmation should replace the airway adjunct to secure an adequate airway. After the fourth shock, the patient presents in the following rhythm. You continue transportation to the emergency department, ensuring good CPR is performed en route. An ACP may administer atropine (1.0 mg).

Cardiac Monitor

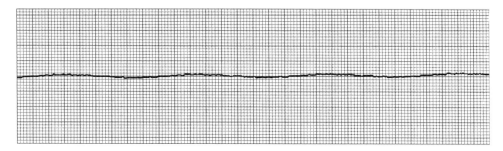

Figure 12.5

Differential Diagnosis

- AMI leading to cardiac arrest.

Test Your Knowledge

1. Why is ASA included in the treatment of this patient?
2. What classifications are the patient's medications?
3. What is the benefit of morphine in the treatment of the patient's chest pain?
4. The skin may be a great indicator of perfusion. What should a paramedic look for in reference to the skin?
5. What is the proper placement for the application of defibrillator pads?
6. What are the methods for confirming endotracheal tube placement in the VSA patient?
7. What ECG is the patient presenting in?

CASE 12.4

You are dispatched at 18:37hrs on a warm May night to 14 Beaver Street, Parry Sound, Ontario, for a man with chest pain. His front door is open when you arrive. You cautiously approach the house, announcing your presence. You hear a male voice from upstairs. You glance upstairs and see a male crouched on the floor. He is pale and tells you he is having chest pain and cannot move. You approach and through conversation learn that the patient's name is Fern Lavigne and he is 55 years old. He tells you that he was upstairs and suddenly felt as though someone had stuck a knife through his chest into his back.

Initial Assessment Findings & Chief Complaint

LOA	Conscious, alert.
A	Patent.
B	Regular, shallow.
C	No radial pulse, but carotid and femoral pulse present.
Wet Check	Unremarkable.
CC	Sharp chest pain radiating to back.

History

S	The patient complains of a sharp pain in his chest and dizziness. He tells you that his legs are very weak and he feels as though he cannot stand.
A	Amitriptyline.
M	doxepin, Flexeril, Tylenol 3, Celebrex, Sectral, Capoten.
P	Work-related back injury two years earlier, MI three years earlier, hypertension.
L	Barbeque at 17:00hrs.
E	Fern says he walked upstairs, went to the bathroom, and when he got up to come down the stairs he had a sudden onset of sharp chest pain radiating to the mid-scapulas. He could not move anymore, sat down, and called 911. He tells you he began sweating profusely and feels as though he has to go to the bathroom again. He has not taken his regular pain medication for two days as he has just returned from a canoe trip where he ran out of Flexeril and Tylenol 3.

Assessment

H/N	No JVD, trachea midline.
Chest	Unremarkable, equal air entry, no adventitious sounds.
ABD	Unremarkable.
Back	Unremarkable.
Pelvis	Stable.
Ext	Lower extremities weak, poor colour with mottling, and no palpable pedal pulses.

Vitals

BP	70/60
P	38, regular
RR	20
Pupils	PERL 4+ mm
GCS	4+5+6=15
BS	n/a
Pulse oximetry	97%
Skin	Pale, diaphoretic

Pain Assessment

O	Sudden onset
P	Just after going to the bathroom
Q	Stabbing, sharp
R	Radiates to mid-scapulas and lower back
S	10/10, worst back pain ever
T	Unrelieved since onset, approximately 30 minutes

Cardiac Monitor

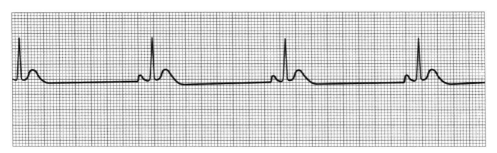

Figure 12.6

Initial Treatment Post Assessment

The patient should be assessed where he is sitting. Oxygen should be administered because of his poor perfusion. Cardiac monitoring should be carried out and a complete set of vitals obtained. The patient should be handled gently and carried to the waiting stretcher by stair-chair or other extrication device. The patient should then be transported without delay to the closest emergency department. An intravenous should be initiated en route, utilizing a large bore IV and run at TKVO. A judgment should be made as to whether this patient should receive a fluid bolus of 20 ml/kg. Constant monitoring of vitals is required throughout transport.

Differential Diagnosis

- Aortic aneurysm.

Test Your Knowledge

1. What cardiac rhythm is the patient presenting with?
2. Why is there lack of circulation and mottling in the lower extremities?
3. What are the classifications of the patient's medications?

4. Why should you be cautious regarding the administration of a fluid bolus with this patient?
5. What are the typical signs and symptoms of an aortic aneurysm?
6. What is the difference between an aortic dissection and an aortic aneurysm?
7. What are the typical signs and symptoms of aortic aneurysms?
8. Why should a large bore IV catheter be used in securing an IV?

Answers
Case 12.1

1. *What is significant about the patient's position when you arrive on scene?*

    The patient is sitting up in bed in an attempt to expand her chest, increasing her tidal volume and alleviating some of her extreme dyspnea.

2. *What are the typical signs and symptoms of congestive heart failure?*

    The typical signs and symptoms of congestive heart failure include:

    Shortness of breath, particularly with exercise
    Coughing, wheezing
    Peripheral edema
    Increased urination
    Weight gain
    Fatigue
    Tachycardia, dysrhythmias

3. *The patient is taking several medications. What are their classifications?*

Altace (ramipril)	– ACE inhibitor
Norvasc (amlodipine)	– Calcium channel blocker
digoxin (Lanoxin)	– Cardiac glycoside
Zestoretic (hydrochlorothiazide, lisinopril)	– Diuretic/ACE inhibitor
NTG (nitroglycerin)	– Peripheral vasodilator
Zoloft (sertraline)	– Selective serotonin reuptake inhibitor (SSRI)
flurbiprofen (Ansaid)	– NSAID
Diamox (acetazolamide)	– Carbonic anhydrase inhibitor

4. *Why do episodes of congestive heart failure occur so frequently in the early morning hours?*

    The majority of CHF patients are on anti-hypertension medications taken once or twice daily. The last usual dose of any anti-hypertensive medication is 18:00hrs. As the patient sleeps, the medication wears off, and blood pressure increases. This leads to nocturnal hypertension and puts stressors on the cardiovascular system, which tends to be weaker than normal. As fluid overloads the system, pulmonary edema develops.

5. *What cardiac rhythm is the patient presenting with?*

    The patient is presenting with an atrial fibrillation.

6. *How does the administration of NTG help this patient?*

    Nitroglycerin administration decreases blood flow to the heart (preload), thus decreasing the work the heart has to do. In patients with pulmonary edema, NTG decreases pressures and increases blood flow because of vasodilation of the pulmonary vasculature.

7. *Why has diuretic therapy become "old school" in the treatment of CHF patients, although it may be beneficial in some instances?*

    Diuretic therapy in hospital has become secondary to positive pressure ventilation through CPAP or BPAP. With positive pressure ventilation, fluids are expelled from the lungs without causing excessive diuresis. In the past, high concentrations of diuretics were utilized, resulting in a fluid and electrolyte imbalance. This necessitated extended hospital stays to enable patients to become hemodynamically stable once again.

8. **Why should the patient not be positioned supine on your stretcher for transport to the emergency department?**

   The patient should not lie supine because of the pulmonary edema and crackles on auscultation. Positioning the patient supine would redistribute the fluid in the lungs, causing more dyspnea and hypoxia and ultimately leading to respiratory failure.

Case 12.2

1. **Why is Stella argumentative when you arrive on scene?**

   As you do not know Stella personally, you cannot determine whether this is simply her personality. However, her response may reflect the fact that she is unaware she has fainted. This is quite common post syncopal episode or post seizure (during the post-ictal period). Other causes of her confusion could include hypoxia and hypoglycemia.

2. **What are the classifications of the patient's medications?**

NTG patch (nitroglycerin)	– Vascular smooth muscle relaxation (transdermal)
Cardizem (diltiazem)	– Calcium channel blocker
Paxil (paroxetine)	– SSRI
Ativan (lorazepam)	– Anxiolytic
Xanax (alprazolam)	– Benzodiazepine
glyburide (Diabeta)	– Oral hypoglycemic
Prevacid (lansoprazole)	– Proton pump inhibitor, H. pylori
Tylenol (acetaminophen)	– Analgesic

3. **What is your interpretation of the patient's ECG?**

   The patient is presenting in a third-degree AV block.

4. **What would be the best way to move the patient from her chair to the stretcher for transport?**

   The patient should be moved with a fore-and-aft lift. She should not be permitted to stand and pivot to the stretcher. The patient may have another syncopal episode brought on by standing.

5. **What may have caused the patient to faint?**

   The patient may have fainted due to coronary insufficiency. With her low heart rate and hypotensive state, supply could not meet demand.

6. **Could Stella be presenting with cardiac insufficiency or an AMI?**

   Stella could be presenting with either cardiac insufficiency or an AMI. She is not perfusing well, based on your observation of her vital signs and skin condition. Stella could also be experiencing a myocardial infarction. A vast majority of elderly patients, particularly females, do not present with chest pain during a heart attack. The most common presentation is an onset of difficulty breathing.

7. **Why is Stella's blood pressure so low?**

   Your patient may be experiencing an inferior MI or may have experienced an MI and may now be in cardiogenic shock. Her heart may be seriously damaged, thus making it a poor forward pump.

Case 12.3

1. **Why is ASA included in the treatment of this patient?**

   ASA inhibits thromboxone A2 and acts as a platelet inhibitor. This prevents platelets from adhering together and increasing the size of the thrombus or adhering to plaque on blood vessel walls. ASA is not an anti-coagulant and does not dissolve clots.

2. **What classifications are the patient's medications?**

Plendil (felodipine)	– Calcium channel blocker
Lopressor (metoprolol)	– Beta blocker
NTG (nitroglycerin)	– Vasodilator
Glucophage (metformin)	– Oral hypoglycemic
Dilantin (phenytoin)	– Anti-convulsant
Naprosyn (naproxen)	– NSAID

3. **What is the benefit of morphine in the treatment of the patient's chest pain?**

   Morphine sulphate is a narcotic analgesic that is administered in the ischemic chest pain patient to reduce pain and aid in the reduction of cardiac preload. It also has sedative properties that may reduce anxiety levels in the patient

4. **The skin is a great indicator of perfusion. What should a paramedic look for in reference to the skin?**

   The paramedic should assess the skin for:

   Colour
   Temperature
   Moisture
   Turgor
   Mobility
   Edema

5. **What is the proper placement for the application of defibrillator pads?**

   One pad should be placed to the right of the upper sternum, just below the clavicle, and the other left of the left nipple in a mid-axillary line.

6. **What are the methods for confirming endotracheal tube placement in the VSA patient?**

   Auscultate for absent breath sounds over the epigastrium
   Auscultate the lung fields for equal bilateral air entry
   Auscultate at the neck for cuff leak
   Visualize the passing through the cords
   Verification of the ETT by an esophageal detector device
   End-tital CO2 monitoring

7. **What ECG is the patient presenting in?**

   The patient is presenting first in a ventricular tachycardia; later, a ventricular fibrillation, and finally an asystole.

Case 12.4

1. **What cardiac rhythm is the patient presenting with?**

   The patient is presenting in a sinus bradycardia.

2. **Why is there lack of circulation and mottling in the lower extremities?**

   There is a lack of peripheral circulation because of the lack of circulating volume and the decrease in blood pressure. The amount of circulating blood and pressure is diminished because of the increased size and volume of the descending aorta.

3. **What are the classifications of the patient's medications?**

doxepin (Sinequan)	– Tricyclic antidepressant
Flexeril (cyclobenzaprine)	– Muscle relaxant
Tylenol 3 (acetaminophen with codeine 30 mg)	– Narcotic analgesic
Celebrex (celecoxib)	– NSAID

Sectral (acebutalol) — Beta blocker
Capoten (captopril) — ACE Inhibitor

4. *Why should you be cautious regarding the administration of a fluid bolus with this patient?*

   The patient's blood pressure is definitely considered hypotensive at 70/60. Although hypotensive, the patient is still alert and his core and brain are perfusing adequately. The addition of a fluid bolus will increase the amount of circulating volume, increasing blood pressure and therefore forcing greater dissection of the aneurysm, worsening the patient's condition. Slow and steady wins the race.

5. *What are the typical signs and symptoms of an aortic aneurysm?*

   The typical signs and symptoms of an aortic aneurysm are:

   Chest pain (tearing or ripping)
   Back pain
   Feeling of fullness without having eaten a large amount
   Nausea
   Vomiting
   Pulsating mass or strong pulse in the abdomen
   Diaphoresis
   Dizziness
   Rapid breathing
   Hypotension
   Tachycardia
   Bradycardia

6. *What is the difference between an aortic dissection and an aortic aneurysm?*

   Aortic dissection is the degeneration of the wall of the aorta, while an aortic aneurysm is a rupture of the aorta itself.

7. *What are the typical causes of aortic aneurysms?*

   The typical causes of aortic aneurysms are atherosclerosis and hypertension. Other causes include blunt trauma or Marfan syndrome.

8. *Why should a large bore IV catheter be used in securing an IV?*

   A large bore IV catheter should be used as it can facilitate administration of blood products as quickly as possible in the emergency department. Blood products require a minimum 18 g catheter.

Chapter 13
Neurology

Many diseases and conditions can cause nervous system disorders. Paramedics should maintain a solid knowledge of the nervous system and its treatments. Every neurological injury and illness, as with other patient presentations, requires a thorough assessment and incident history. Neurological disorders involve many presentations and complaints, ranging from headaches to altered levels of consciousness. Paramedic treatment involves maintaining adequate oxygenation and determining possible causes of any altered level of consciousness, e.g., hypoglycemia. Although most care for neurological patients is supportive, some may require care as soon as possible after assessment to prevent progressive or permanent damage. Early treatment for potential stroke patients requires the development of a timeline and rapid transport to a stroke centre.

CASE 13.1

You are dispatched to St. Luke's Church in Old Crow, Yukon, on a cold winter Sunday morning for a possible unconscious patient. On arrival, you are directed to the centre of a pew in the middle of the church, where an elderly man is being supported by several people. Tom, who is with his 80-year-old father Charlie, tells you that they were listening to the sermon when his father fell sideways. Tom tried to talk to him, but his father would not reply and now appears to be staring away to the right. Tom reports that his father has a bad heart, high blood pressure, and diabetes.

Initial Assessment Findings & Chief Complaint

LOA	Conscious but appears confused.
A	Patent with saliva drooling from the left side.
B	Regular at 14.
C	Strong and irregular radial pulses.
Wet Check	Unremarkable.
CC	Altered level of awareness, sudden onset of weakness, and unable to speak.

History

S	Sudden onset of left-sided weakness and the inability to speak.
A	atenolol.
M	moexipril, digoxin, Aldactone, Ansaid, Tofranil, Humulin N, Humulin R
P	Hypertension, diabetes, atrial fibrillation.
L	Breakfast.
E	The patient was in church and suddenly fell to one side and was unable to speak.

Assessment

H/N	Unremarkable.
Chest	Equal air entry bilaterally with no adventitious sounds.
ABD	Soft/non-tender.
Back	Unremarkable.
Pelvis	Stable.
Ext	Right upper and lower extremities have equal strength and mobility while the left upper and lower extremities have notable decreased strength.

Vitals

BP	240/118
P	150, irregular
RR	16 full volume
Pupils	L: PERL 3+ mm
	R: PERL 4+ mm slow
GCS	4+1+5=10
BS	5.8 mmol/l
Pulse oximetry	96%
Skin	Warm, dry

Pain Assessment

O	n/a
P	n/a
Q	n/a
R	n/a
S	n/a
T	n/a

Cardiac Monitor

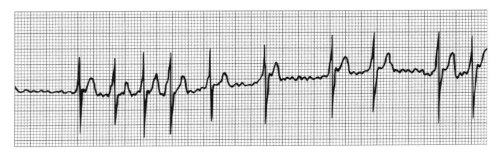

Figure 13.1

Initial Treatment Post Assessment

The patient should be assessed and a complete set of vitals obtained including a blood glucometry. ECG interpretation should be completed. The patient should be supported and administered oxygen via a high concentration mask. A determination of the actual time of the onset of symptoms should be made based on information obtained from the son. The patient should be transported in a semi-sitting position with slight elevation on the right side to facilitate drainage of saliva from the patient's mouth. An intravenous can be established en route to a hospital and run at TKVO.

Differential Diagnosis

- Possible cerebral vascular accident (CVA).

Test Your Knowledge

1. What are typical signs and symptoms of a stroke?
2. What are the two categories of strokes?
3. What is the definitive treatment for an embolic stroke?

4. What classifications of medications is Tom's father being prescribed?
5. What is the difference between a stroke and a transient ischemic attack (TIA)?
6. What ECG rhythm is the patient presenting with?
7. The time from the onset of symptoms to the possible treatment of an embolic stroke with fibrinolytics must be less than ____ hours.
8. If a patient is found beside his or her bed in the morning and a stroke is suspected, would the patient be a candidate for a possible stroke code?

CASE 13.2

You are dispatched at 17:43hrs to the Family Restaurant, 70 Coral Street, Emo, Ontario, for a patient in possible seizure. On arrival, you find an 18-year-old woman lying on the floor of the restaurant with a young man sitting beside her. The woman appears to be sleeping or resting on her side. The young man, Marty, tells you that Brenda had a seizure lasting approximately one minute. He describes the seizure as total upper and lower body jerking. She stopped just before you arrived on scene. Marty has a wet facecloth on Brenda's forehead. He tells you that she has a history of epilepsy but has been trying to wean herself off her meds because she has not had a seizure in five years. He just started going out with her three months ago.

Initial Assessment Findings & Chief Complaint

LOA	Responds to loud verbal stimuli by looking at you.
A	Patent.
B	Full volume at 12.
C	Strong radial pulse.
Wet Check	Incontinent of urine.
CC	Possible seizure.

History

S	Patient had a witnessed seizure lasting approximately one minute.
A	Tegretol.
M	phenobarbital, phenytoin.
P	Epilepsy.
L	Halfway through lunch.
E	Brenda was eating lunch when she told her boyfriend she felt funny. She then began to have a total full body seizure. Marty lowered her to the floor and supported her head. The staff at the restaurant called 911 immediately.

Assessment

H/N	No JVD, trachea midline, no obvious trauma.
Chest	Unremarkable, equal air entry bilaterally.
ABD	Unremarkable.
Back	Unremarkable.
Pelvis	Stable.
Ext	Unremarkable, equal strength and mobility bilaterally

Vitals

BP	116/80
P	75 strong and regular
RR	12 full volume
Pupils	PERL 3+ mm
GCS	4+3+4=11
BS	6.8 mmol/l
Pulse oximetry	98%
Skin	Warm, dry

Pain Assessment

O	n/a
P	n/a
Q	n/a
R	n/a
S	n/a
T	n/a

Cardiac Monitor

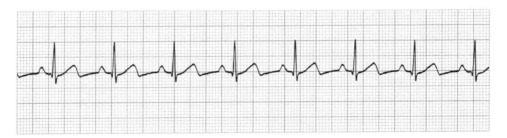

Figure 13.2

Initial Treatment Post Assessment

An initial assessment of the patient should be completed, including a good visual of the patient's airway since she was eating at the time of the seizure. A complete set of vitals, including blood glucometry, should be obtained. The patient should have a cardiac monitor applied and an ECG interpretation should be performed. Oxygen via a high concentration mask should be administered. An intravenous should also be initiated and run at TKVO. The patient should be transported in a semi-prone position to the waiting ambulance.

Just as you are loading Brenda into the ambulance, she has a full tonic-clonic (generalized motor) seizure.

Treatment Continued

You and your partner continue loading the patient into the ambulance while your partner controls her swinging head, preventing it from banging into the wall of the ambulance cupboards. After approximately 40 seconds, Brenda's seizure becomes confined to her upper and lower extremities with minimal head movement. An ACP should now slowly administer diazepam or lorazepam via IV to stop the seizure. The patient's airway should be assessed, and if perfusion is inadequate or the seizure continues, ventilation with a BVM should be attempted. Transport to a local emergency centre should be expedited after the administration of the medication. Once the seizure stops, the patient's airway should be reassessed for secretions or vomitus. A repeat blood glucometry should also be obtained. Oxygen should be administered en route.

Differential Diagnosis

- Seizure.

Test Your Knowledge

1. What phases are associated with a tonic-clonic or grand mal seizure?
2. What is an aura?
3. What ECG is the patient presenting with?
4. What classifications are the patient's medications?
5. What is the most common cause of status epilepticus in adults?
6. What classifications of medications are diazepam or lorazepam, used in the treatment of seizures in a pre-hospital setting?
7. Why might a patient be confused following a seizure?

CASE 13.3

You are dispatched to West Edmonton Mall for a 63-year-old female who is complaining of dizziness and unable to walk. As you approach, you observe the patient supporting herself on a bench with her arm. You introduce yourself and she acknowledges you, speaking with an atypical-sounding hoarse voice. She introduces herself as Rashad. She tells you that she was walking in the mall when she suddenly became very dizzy and weak on her left side. She adds that she feels as though she might fall over because of her unsteady gait, and says that everything looks tilted. You notice her eyes are moving quickly from side to side.

Initial Assessment Findings & Chief Complaint

LOA	Conscious and alert.
A	Patent.
B	Full volume.
C	Strong radial pulses, irregular.
Wet Check	Unremarkable.
CC	Unexplained vertigo and weakness.

History

S	Dizziness and weakness.
A	Sulpha drugs.
M	Mevacor, Ativan, Celebrex, Feldene.
P	High cholesterol, arthritis.
L	Just ate at the food court.
E	The patient was walking and became weak on the left side and dizzy. She denies pain.

Assessment

H/N	No JVD, trachea midline, numbness in the right side of her face. No facial drooping noted.
Chest	Equal air entry bilaterally without adventitious sounds.
ABD	Soft/non-tender.
Back	Unremarkable.
Pelvis	Stable.
Ext	Weakness in left upper and lower extremities, while right-sided extremities appear normal. Good mobility bilaterally.

Vitals

Pain Assessment

BP	186/110	O	n/a
P	150 irregular	P	n/a
RR	14 full volume	Q	n/a
Pupils	PERL 3+ mm	R	n/a
GCS	4+5+6=15	S	n/a
BS	4.6 mmol/l	T	n/a
Pulse oximetry	97%		
Skin	Warm, dry		

Cardiac Monitor

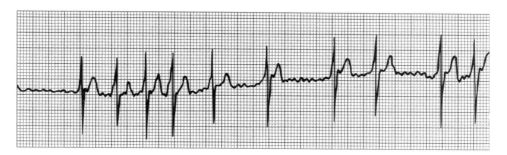

Figure 13.3

Initial Treatment Post Assessment

The patient should be assessed and vitals obtained, including a blood glucometry. Cardiac monitoring should be performed. Oxygen via a nasal cannula at 2–6 lpm should be administered. The patient should be transported to the hospital with supportive care.

En route, there is no change in the patient's condition, although she is becoming more nauseated and thinks she may vomit. Her vitals signs remain consistent.

Treatment Continued

To relieve the patient's nausea, an ACP may initiate intravenous dimenhydrinate.

Differential Diagnosis

- Wallenberg's syndrome.

Test Your Knowledge

1. What is the cause of Wallenberg's syndrome?
2. What is your interpretation of the patient's ECG?
3. What are the signs and symptoms of Wallenberg's syndrome?
4. What classifications are the patient's medications?
5. What cranial nerves may be affected by this condition?
6. What is another name for Wallenberg's syndrome?

122 Division 2 Medical Emergencies

CASE 13.4

You are dispatched to 14 Bryden Avenue, Halifax, for a 43-year-old female who has had a headache for the past five hours. On arrival you are met by her husband Myron, who tells you that his wife, Tawneysia, was driven home early from work by a friend due to a severe headache. He reports that she is under a huge amount of stress at work as a deadline for a job is fast approaching. She has had headaches in the past, but nothing this severe. He tells you that she had a Tylenol 2 at the office but the headache didn't go away. She has vomited once since her husband has been home. As you head toward the dark bedroom, you hear sniffling; she appears to be crying. Myron tells you that his wife can tolerate a lot of pain, so she must be hurting.

Initial Assessment Findings and Chief Complaint

LOA	Conscious and alert.
A	Patent.
B	Regular and full volume.
C	Strong radial pulse.
Wet Check	Unremarkable.
CC	Headache.

History

S	Throbbing left-sided headache.
A	None.
M	Tylenol 2, Zoloft, NicoDerm patch.
P	Depression, headaches.
L	Lunch at work.
E	Tawneysia states that she was at work and started getting a pain in the left side of her head. She took a Tylenol 2 thinking it would make the pain subside. Instead, the pain progressed to the point of throbbing when she kept her eyes open. After vomiting at work, she was driven home and lay down in her bedroom.

Assessment

H/N	No JI21VD, trachea midline. Pain in the left side of the patient's head with a tender scalp.
Chest	Unremarkable, with equal air entry bilaterally
ABD	Soft/non-tender.
Back	Unremarkable.
Pelvis	Stable.
Ext	Unremarkable with equal strength.

Vitals

BP	126/86
P	73, slightly irregular
RR	16 regular
Pupils	PERL 3+ mm
GCS	4+5+6=15
BS	n/a
Pulse oximetry	100%
Skin	Warm, moist

Pain Assessment

O	Gradually
P	While working at the computer
Q	Throbbing
R	Front to back left side only
S	10/10
T	5 hours

Cardiac Monitor

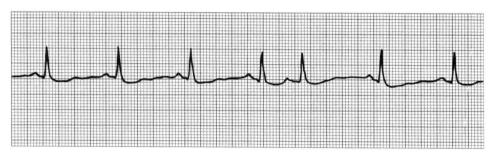

Figure 13.4

Initial Treatment Post Assessment

The patient should be assessed and vitals should be obtained, including SPO2, blood sugar, and ECG interpretation. The patient should receive oxygen via a high concentration mask. An intravenous should be initiated and infused at TKVO. The patient should be transported in a position of comfort with a quiet environment and dimmed interior lights. Analgesics should not be administered to this patient until a differential diagnosis can be confirmed.

En route, the patient settles and falls asleep.

Differential Diagnosis

- Migraine headache.

Test Your Knowledge

1. What is significant about the patient's position when you arrive on scene?
2. What are typical signs and symptoms of a migraine headache?
3. What are the differences between migraine, cluster, and tension headaches?
4. What ECG is the patient presenting with?

5. What are the classifications of the patient's medications?
6. What else could be causing the patient's headache?

Answers
Case 13.1

1. **What are typical signs and symptoms of a stroke?**

    The signs and symptoms of a stroke may include:
    - Headache
    - Facial flaccidity or drooping
    - Confusion
    - Agitation
    - Dysphasia or aphasia
    - Dysphagia
    - Dysarthria
    - Hemiparesis
    - Hemiplegia
    - Unsteady gait
    - Vertigo
    - Altered level of consciousness

2. **What are the two categories of strokes?**

    The two categories of strokes are embolic and hemorrhagic.

3. **What is the definitive treatment for an embolic stroke?**

    The definitive treatment for an embolic stroke is thrombolytic therapy; for example, with the use of a tissue plasminogen activator (tPA).

4. **What classifications of medications is Tom's father being prescribed?**

Medication	Classification
moexipril (Univasc)	– ACE Inhibitor
digoxin (Lanoxin)	– Cardiac glycoside
Aldactone (spironolactone)	– Potassium-sparing diuretic
Ansaid (flurbiprofen)	– NSAID
Tofranil (imipramine)	– Antidepressant
Humulin N (insulin)	– Intermediate acting insulin
Humulin R (insulin)	– Rapid acting insulin

5. **What is the difference between a stroke and a transient ischemic attack (TIA)?**

    The distinguishing characteristic of a TIA is that the stroke-like symptoms will usually resolve within 24 hours. Unlike a stroke, once the symptoms have resolved, there will be no residual neurological damage.

6. **What ECG rhythm is the patient presenting with?**

    The patient is presenting with an atrial fibrillation.

7. **The time from the onset of symptoms to the possible treatment of an embolic stroke with fibrinolytics must be less than ____ hours.**

    The time from the onset of symptoms to the possible treatment of an embolic stroke with fibrinolytics must be less than **three** hours.

8. **If a patient is found beside his or her bed in the morning and a stroke is suspected, would the patient be a candidate for a possible stroke code?**

    Since the actual time of onset cannot be determined, such a patient would not be suitable for treatment according to a stroke code, which is a protocol for the early treatment of suspected stroke patients.

Case 13.2

1. ***What phases are associated with a tonic-clonic or grand mal seizure?***

    The phases associated with a tonic-clonic, generalized, or grand mal seizure include:
    Aura
    Loss of consciousness
    Tonic phase
    Hypertonic phase
    Clonic phase
    Post seizure
    Post-ictal

2. ***What is an aura?***

    An aura is a sensation preceding a seizure. Auras may include taste, auditory, visual, or olfactory hallucinations. Not all seizures are preceded by auras.

3. ***What ECG is the patient presenting with?***

    The patient is presenting with a normal sinus rhythm.

4. ***What classifications are the patient's medications?***

    Phenobarbital (phenobarbital) — Barbituate
    phenytoin (Dilantin) — Anti-convulsant

5. ***What is the most common cause of status epilepticus in adults?***

    The most common cause of status epilepticus is poor medication compliance or failing to take medications. Patients may go seizure-free for years while taking medication, feel they no longer need to take it, and begin to reduce the dosage. As the dosage is decreased, the incidence of seizures returns.

6. ***What classifications of medications are diazepam or lorazepam, used in the treatment of seizures in a pre-hospital setting?***

    Diazepam (Valium) and lorazepam (Ativan), used in the treatment of seizures, are both considered benzodiazepines.

7. ***Why might a patient be confused following a seizure?***

    Hypoxia may cause a patient to become confused after a seizure as he or she enters the post-ictal phase. During a seizure, due to extreme muscular rigidity, there is a lack of adequate respiration. The patient becomes hypoxic and will require time afterward to regain the full awareness of his or her surroundings. Supplemental oxygen administration aids in recovery.

Case 13.3

1. ***What is Wallenberg's syndrome caused by?***

    Wallenberg's syndrome is caused by an occlusion of the vertebral or posterior inferior cerebellar artery (PICA) or one of its branches, which supply the lower brain stem. This results in sensory, sympathetic, and cerebellar disturbances.

2. ***What is your interpretation of the patient's ECG?***

    The patient is presenting in an atrial fibrillation.

3. ***What are the signs and symptoms of Wallenberg's syndrome?***

    Signs and symptoms of Wallenberg's syndrome include:
    Nausea
    Vomiting
    Ipsilateral ataxia
    Muscular hyertonicity
    Pain

　　　　Facial paresthesia
　　　　Homolateral nystagmus
　　　　Dysphasia
　　　　Dysphagia
　　　　Dysphonia
　　　　Hiccups

4. **What classifications are the patient's medications?**

Mevacor (lovastatin)	– Lipid metabolism regulator
Ativan (lorazepam)	– Benzodiazepine, anxiolytic
Celebrex (celecoxib)	– NSAID
Feldene (piroxicam)	– NSAID

5. **What cranial nerves may be affected by this condition?**

   Cranial nerves V, IX, X, and XII may be affected.

6. **What is another name for Wallenberg's syndrome?**

   Another name for Wallenberg's syndrome is lateral medullary plate syndrome.

Case 13.4

1. **What is significant about the patient's position when you arrive on scene?**

   The patient is lying in her bedroom in the dark. This indicates that she may be photosensitive. She is motionless, indicating that her headache is provoked by movement.

2. **What are typical signs and symptoms of a migraine headache?**

   Typical signs of a migraine headache include:
   　　Usually gradual onset
   　　Typically unilateral
   　　Usually pulsating and worsened by physical activity
   　　Nausea
   　　Vomiting
   　　Photosensitivity
   　　Phonophobia
   　　May be preceded by an aura

3. **What are the differences between migraine, cluster, and tension headaches?**

Cluster headache:	A series of one-sided headaches
	Intense
	May cause nasal congestion, drooping eyelid, watery eyes
	Most occur in men
Migraine headache:	Most occur in women
	Intense or throbbing pain
	Photosensitivity and phonosensitivity
	Usually unilateral
Tension headache:	Morning headaches that get worse throughout the day
	Dull, achy pain
	Pressure in neck and head

4. **What ECG is the patient presenting with?**

   The patient is presenting in a normal sinus rhythm with PACs.

5. *What are the classifications of the patient's medications?*

   Tylenol 2 (acetaminophen with codeine)   – Narcotic analgesic
   Zoloft (sertraline)   – Antidepressant
   NicoDerm patch (nicotine)   – Smoking cessation patch

6. *What else could be causing the patient's headache?*

   The patient is also using a NicoDerm patch to aid in breaking her smoking habit. Signs and symptoms of nicotine overdose include several of the symptoms the patient is presenting with, including:
   - Sweats
   - Nausea
   - Vomiting
   - Headache
   - Dizziness
   - Visual disturbances

Chapter 14
Endocrinology

Unlike the nervous system, the endocrine system controls the body through hormones that affect processes in body systems. The majority of endocrine emergencies involve complications of diabetes mellitus. However, other issues involving the endocrine system may also be routinely exposed during the assessment of a patient or when obtaining a patient's medical history. Most endocrine conditions are not life-threatening, but may have an impact on other illnesses. Hypoglycemia and hyperglycemia are the most urgent diabetic emergencies and can be treated in the pre-hospital field. Early detection and intervention by a paramedic can have a significant impact on a patient's outcome.

CASE 14.1

At 10:30hrs on a snowy December day in Maple Ridge, British Columbia, you are dispatched to a residence for a female who is generally unwell. On arrival, you are greeted by the patient's husband and told that his wife, Nancy, has not been feeling well for the past four days. The husband takes you to their bedroom on the second floor. As you enter, you see a moderately obese woman who appears to be in her sixties lying propped up in bed. She seems lethargic and distant as you approach.

Initial Assessment Findings & Chief Complaint

LOA	Appears confused, distant.
A	Patent.
B	Regular and full volume.
C	Strong, rapid, irregular radial pulses.
Wet Check	Unremarkable.
CC	The patient is complaining of being dry and always thirsty. She has also had an upset stomach and has been vomiting for the past two days. She tells you she just wants to sleep.

History

S	Flushed, dry mouth, and very thirsty with vomiting for the past two days.
A	Peanut butter, latex, cats, dogs.
M	Lasix, Lipitor, glyburide, amoxicillin.
P	Hypertension, high cholesterol, diabetes, urinary tract infection (recent).
L	Supper last night, although she managed to keep only a small amount of food down.
E	The patient has been inactive and lethargic for the past four days.

Assessment

H/N	Unremarkable.
Chest	Clear x4, no adventitious sounds.
ABD	Soft visceral pain on palpation.
Back	Unremarkable.
Pelvis	Stable.
Ext	Class II peripheral edema to ankles.

Vitals

BP	130/100
P	150, irregular
RR	20 regular
Pupils	PERL 4 mm
GCS	4+4+5=13
BS	34.0 mmol/l
Pulse oximetry	96%
Skin	Warm, dry

Pain Assessment

O	gradual
P	n/a
Q	dull
R	none
S	6/10
T	2 days

Cardiac Monitor

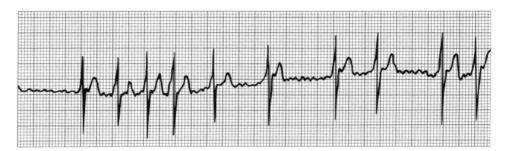

Figure 14.1

Initial Treatment Post Assessment

The patient should be assessed for her mental status and possible reason for confusion. Oxygen via nasal cannula at 36% should be administered to maintain a pulse oximetry of 98-100%. Blood sugar reveals a glucometry of 34.0 mmol/l. An IV should be established and administered at TKVO. If protocols dictate, insulin or an insulin drip may be administered. The patient should be extricated from upstairs, which may require additional resources due to her weakness.

En route to the hospital, the patient has an approximately 45-second tonic-clonic seizure and remains post-ictal.

Treatment Continued

Appropriate assessment of the patient's airway should be completed in her post-ictal state. A nasopharyngeal airway should be inserted to help maintain airway patency. Should SPO2 and her respiratory rate fall, respirations should be supported. Advanced airway manoeuvres should be withheld until the outcome of the post-ictal state is determined. If the patient remains unconscious, then a combitube or intubation could be initiated. Should the patient seize again, intravenous midazolam, diazepam, or lorazepam should be administered. A repeat blood glucometry should also be performed.

Differential Diagnosis

- Hyperglycemic Hyperosmolar Nonketotic Acidosis (HHNK).
- Seizure caused by a hyperglycemic state.

Test Your Knowledge

1. What cardiac rhythm is the patient presenting in?
2. What classifications are the patient's medications?
3. What conditions contribute to Hyperglycemic Hyperosmolar Nonketonic Acidosis (HHNK)?
4. What are the signs and symptoms of HHNK?
5. Why is the mortality rate for HHNK greater than that for diabetic ketoacidosis?
6. Why are Kussmaul's respirations absent with HHNK?
7. What may have contributed to Nancy's hyperglycemic emergency?

CASE 14.2

At 16:00hrs you are dispatched to 1350 Mountview Crescent, Gunnar, Saskatchewan, for a possible violent patient. You proceed and join up with local police as you pull into the driveway of a quiet neighbourhood. On arrival, you are met by the patient's mother and told that her 16-year-old son Dan is punching walls and throwing CDs around his room. She tells you that when she tried to talk to him, he pushed her away. She says, "He is a diabetic and has never acted this way before." She is very upset and does not want her son to be hurt or arrested as he is "a good kid." In his bedroom, Dan is partially clothed and urinating while standing on his bed. Police officers wait momentarily before they tackle and physically restrain him on the bed. You are now able to begin your assessment.

Initial Assessment Findings and Chief Complaint

LOA	Patient appears confused and scared with your presence and that of the local police.
A	Airway appears patent, since Dan is screaming at you to leave him alone.
B	Regular and full although tachypneic.
C	Strong radial pulses.
Wet Check	Urine on his underwear and on the bed.
CC	Abnormal behaviour, violent tendencies.

History

S	Violent and abnormal behaviour toward himself and those who approach him after returning from playing basketball with a group of friends.
A	codeine, environmental.
M	Humulin L, Humulin R, Allegra.
P	Diabetes (recently diagnosed).
L	Lunch.
E	Dan was playing basketball for approximately 45 minutes, came home, and appeared confused and angry. He began punching walls and breaking articles in his room. His mother denies drug use by Dan. She could not control him so she called 911.

Assessment

H/N	Unremarkable.
Chest	Unremarkable with equal air entry absent of adventitious sounds.
ABD	Soft/non-tender.
Back	Unremarkable.
Pelvis	Stable.
Ext	Minor abrasions on the knuckles of both hands.

Vitals

BP	110/70
P	150, regular
RR	20 shallow
Pupils	PERL 4+ mm
GCS	4+3+6=13
BS	2.2 mmol/l
Pulse oximetry	99%
Skin	Pale, diaphoretic

Pain Assessment

O	n/a
P	n/a
Q	n/a
R	n/a
S	n/a
T	n/a

Cardiac Monitor

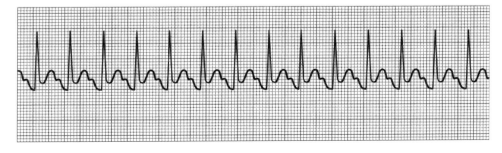

Figure 14.2

Initial Treatment Post Assessment

The initial assessment should be completed while Dan is being restrained. Dan's violence is not normal behaviour for him, so he should be told what you will be doing and why. Oxygen saturation should be conducted to rule out hypoxia as a cause of his behaviour. Appropriate vitals should be obtained, including a blood glucometry. Once completed, an intravenous should be attempted. If an IV cannot be established, the patient should be given Glucagon IM for his hypoglycemia. If an IV can be initiated, 1 amp of D50W should be administered, as the patient is hypoglycemic. Repeat blood glucometry should be performed once Dan has settled and becomes more alert.

Dan becomes alert and tells you he started feeling funny at the court and just wanted to get home. He does not remember anything that happened after arriving home. He is apologetic and does not want to go to the hospital. You advise him to have something to eat and of the importance of maintaining an insulin-intake balance, especially when playing sports or increasing physical activity. He signs your appropriate call reports and you leave the scene.

Differential Diagnosis

- Hypoglycemic emergency.

Test Your Knowledge

1. What is significant about Dan's violent tendencies, and what may be causing this behaviour?
2. What are the classifications of Dan's medications?
3. What are the typical signs and symptoms of hypoglycemia?
4. What is a contraindication for the administration of glucagon?
5. What are possible causes of hypoglycemia?
6. What are possible long-term complications of diabetes?
7. Does hypoglycemia have a rapid or slow onset?
8. Is hypoglycemia a true medical emergency?
9. What ECG rhythm is the patient presenting with?

CASE 14.3

You are working a quiet day shift in Grosses Coques, NS, when a call comes in for an unconscious 45-year-old lying on the sidewalk outside Frenchy's. As you pull up to the scene, a store employee meets you and reports that Ruby, who is well-known to all, was sitting on the bench and suddenly slouched over. The staff lowered her to the ground and called 911.

Initial Assessment Findings & Chief Complaint

LOA	Unconscious.
A	Appears patent, fruity breath.
B	Snoring respirations.
C	Strong radial pulses present.
Wet Check	Incontinent of urine.
CC	Unconscious NYD.

History

S	Patient is lying semi-prone unconscious on the sidewalk.
A	CNO.
M	Diabenese, Cardizem SR, Tylenol 2, ibuprofen, all found in purse beside patient.
P	MedicAlert bracelet: diabetes, hypertension.
L	CNO.
E	As observed by store staff members, the patient was sitting on a bench for approximately 30 minutes prior to slouching over. The staff assumed that she was sleeping while she waited for someone inside the store. When they could not wake her, they called 911.

Assessment

H/N	No JVD, trachea midline, mild cyanosis of lips/ears.
Chest	Unremarkable, equal snoring respirations, clear bilaterally.
ABD	Soft/non-tender.
Back	Unremarkable.
Pelvis	Stable.
Ext	No trauma noted, mild cyanosis in fingertips.

Vitals

Pain Assessment

BP	100/60	O	n/a
P	130	P	n/a
RR	16, deep, air hunger	Q	n/a
Pupils	PERL 4 mm slow to react	R	n/a
GCS	1+1+1=3	S	n/a
BS	24 mmol/l	T	n/a
Pulse oximetry	92%		
Skin	Warm, dry		

Cardiac Monitor

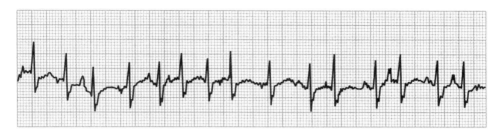

Figure 14.3

Initial Treatment Post Assessment

The patient requires immediate airway management and ventilation to prevent hypoxia and to help with the expulsion of excessive carbon dioxide. The patient should be placed supine on the stretcher, an OPA should be inserted, and ventilation with a BVM should be initiated. Blood glucometry should confirm hypoglycemia. Cardiac monitoring should be completed and maintained throughout transport to a medical facility. An IV should be initiated and infused at TKVO. An ACP should perform endotracheal intubation to secure the airway and reduce the risk of aspiration. If it is within the medic's scope of practice, insulin can be administered to correct the patient's insulin level before advanced airway management is performed.

Differential Diagnosis

- Diabetic ketoacidosis.

Test Your Knowledge

1. What are common causes of diabetic ketoacidosis (DKA)?
2. What medications are related to your patient's endocrine system?
3. What are the classifications of the patient's other medications?
4. What ECG rhythm is the patient presenting with?
5. What are signs and symptoms of DKA?
6. Is the onset of DKA slow or rapid?
7. Why does the patient have a fruity smell on her breath?
8. Does this patient require emergency transport?

Answers

Case 14.1

1. *What cardiac rhythm is the patient presenting in?*

    The patient is presenting in atrial fibrillation, which is not usually caused by a diabetic emergency and may be an underlying rhythm the patient is being treated for.

2. **What classifications are the patient's medications?**

   Lasix (furosemide) — Loop diuretic
   Lipitor (atorvastatin) — Lipid metabolism regulator
   glyburide (Diabeta) — Oral hypoglycemic
   Amoxicillin (Amoxil) — Antibiotic

3. **What conditions contribute to Hyperglycemic Hyperosmolar Nonketonic Acidosis (HHNK)?**

   The following conditions contribute to HHNK: infections, dialysis, high-osmolarity feeding supplements, and certain medications. The incidence of HHNK is usually associated with type II diabetes.

4. **What are the signs and symptoms of HHNK?**

   The typical signs and symptoms associated with HHNK are:

   Rapid pulse
   Normal to low blood pressure
   Normal breathing absent of breath odours
   Polyuria
   Polydipsia
   Polyphagia
   Warm, dry skin and mucous membranes
   Normal vision

5. **Why is the mortality rate of HHNK greater than that of diabetic ketoacidosis?**

   The mortality rate of HHNK is higher than that of diabetic ketoacidosis because of the lack of early signs that would prompt a patient's attention. HHNK usually affects the elderly and may have a mortality rate of 40–70 percent.

6. **Why are Kussmaul's respirations absent with HHNK?**

   Kussmaul's respirations are absent in a patient suffering from HHNK as there is adequate insulin to allow some glucose to enter cells. Because there is no breakdown of fats and proteins for energy, there is an absence of ketone production from pyruvate and byproducts of metabolism.

7. **What may have contributed to Nancy's hyperglycemic emergency?**

   Nancy is on a broad-spectrum antibiotic for a bacterial infection. This may have contributed to her condition. Further investigation and questioning may give more insight as to why and what she was being treated for.

Case 14.2

1. **What is significant about Dan's violent tendencies, and what may be causing this behaviour?**

   Dan's atypical behaviour is caused by a decrease in blood sugar levels in his brain. As this progresses, Dan may be susceptible to a hypoglycemic seizure.

2. **What are the classifications of Dan's medications?**

   Humulin L (insulin lente) — Human biosynthetic intermediate-acting insulin
   Humulin R (insulin regular) — Human biosynthetic rapid-acting insulin
   Allegra (fexofenadine HCL) — Histamine H1-receptor antagonist

3. **What are the typical signs and symptoms of hypoglycemia?**

   The typical signs and symptoms of hypoglycemia include cold and clammy skin, weakness, lack of coordination, headache, irritability, agitated behaviour, decreased mental function, drooling, and diplopia progressing to unconsciousness and/or coma. The patient may present with normal vital signs.

4. **What is a contraindication for the administration of glucagon?**

   A contraindication for the administration of glucagon is pheochromocytoma, a rare adrenal gland tumor. Glucagon can stimulate the tumor to release catecholamines, which may result in a sudden increase in blood pressure similar to a sympathetic response.

5. **What are possible causes of hypoglycemia?**

   The possible causes of hypoglycemia are usually related to an imbalance of sugar intake and insulin. This occurs when the patient administers their normal insulin dosage and does not eat, administers too much insulin, or administers their normal dosage and is involved in excessive exercise or physical activity. In Dan's situation, he administered his normal insulin and ate lunch, but then played basketball for 45 minutes, thereby depleting his sugar stores.

6. **What are possible long-term complications of diabetes?**

   Long-term complications of diabetes can include vascular disease, diabetic retinopathy, glaucoma, and diabetic neuropathy.

7. **Does hypoglycemia have a rapid or slow onset?**

   In contrast to diabetic ketoacidosis, hypoglycemia usually occurs quickly. Any alterations in blood glucose levels affecting glucose intake and insulin administration can cause a change in mental status without warning.

8. **Is hypoglycemia a true medical emergency?**

   Hypoglycemia is a true emergency, as brain cells can be permanently damaged by the lack of glucose. The brain can adapt to use fats as an energy source, but this can take hours. The switch to this form of metabolism cannot correct any permanent damage to the brain caused by the lack of available glucose.

9. **What ECG is the patient presenting in?**

   The patient is presenting in a sinus tachycardia.

Case 14.3

1. **What are common causes of diabetic ketoacidosis (DKA)?**

   The common causes of DKA include physiological stressors, such as an infection blocking insulin effects and potentiating glucagon's effects, and cessation of insulin injections.

2. **What medications are related to your patient's endocrine system?**

   Diabenese (chlorpropamide) – Oral hypoglycemic

3. **What are the classifications of the patient's other medications?**

   Tylenol 2 (acetaminophen-codeine compound) – Narcotic analgesic
   ibuprofen (Motrin) – Non-steroidal anti-inflammatory
   Cardizem (diltiazem HCL) – Calcium channel blocker, antianginal

4. **What ECG rhythm is the patient presenting with?**

   The patient is presenting with a multifocal atrial tachycardia.

5. **What are signs and symptoms of DKA?**

   Polyuria, polydipsia
   Abdominal pain
   Tachycardia
   Hypotension
   Warm, dry skin

Kussmaul's respirations
Possible fruity odour on breath
Nausea/vomiting
Decreased mental status or coma

6. *Is the onset of DKA slow or rapid?*

   The onset of DKA is usually slow, lasting 14–24 hours, in comparison to hypoglycemia, which usually has a rapid onset.

7. *Why does the patient have a fruity smell to her breath?*

   Profound hyperglycemia exists because of a lack of insulin in the body. When insulin cannot enter the cells, gluconeogenesis compounds the problem. The body then metabolizes fat for energy and produces the byproducts pyruvate and ketones. This leads to a reduction in pH, or acidosis. The compensatory mechanism for a metabolic acidotic state is the respiratory system. Breathing becomes rapid and deep to expel excessive acids in the form of carbon dioxide. The fruity smell is a product of blood acetone expelled through the lungs.

8. *Does this patient require emergency transport?*

   This patient requires aggressive intervention to reverse the acidotic state she is presenting with, and rapid transport to a nearby medical facility.

Chapter 15
Allergies and Anaphylaxis

Allergic reactions, although uncommon, present in a rapid fashion that can be detrimental if intervention by paramedics is not prompt. Anaphylaxis can develop within seconds and cause death minutes after exposure to an allergen. It can progress to bronchoconstriction, airway edema, peripheral vasodilation, and hypoxia. Food tends to be the most common cause of anaphylaxis, but insects, medicines, and even latex can cause a reaction. The goals of the paramedic are to reverse the effects of this process and improve perfusion. The primary drug used in the treatment of anaphylaxis is epinephrine. As a supplement to epinephrine, antihistamines and bronchodilators are routinely administered. Early recognition and intervention are key to successful treatment.

CASE 15.1

You are dispatched at 13:00hrs to 45 Railway Avenue, Drumheller, Alberta, for a possible respiratory arrest. As you pull up to the building, you realize it is your family dentist's office. You are met by the dental hygienist as you enter and are directed toward the dentist, who is administering oxygen to a patient via a simple face mask. The patient appears to be having extreme difficulty breathing. Dr. Chabot reports that he had just frozen the patient with Xylocaine and was about to proceed with a routine filling. The patient, Brianna, who is 18 years old, appears to be quite scared. Dr. Chabot tells you that Brianna's chart does not indicate any allergies to anesthetics.

Initial Assessment Findings & Chief Complaint

LOA	Slightly confused, but responds to questions.
A	Appears patent.
B	Shallow and laboured at approximately 36.
C	Strong radial pulse present.
Wet Check	Unremarkable.
CC	Respiratory distress.

History

S	Complains of acute onset of respiratory difficulty.
A	Sulpha drugs.
M	Birth control pills.
P	None.
L	Breakfast.
E	The patient was given a freezing for a dental procedure and five minutes later began experiencing difficulty breathing and a tightness in her neck and chest.

Assessment

H/N	No JVD, trachea midline. Patient complains of difficulty swallowing and a swollen tongue.
Chest	Urticaria present in upper chest, expiratory wheezing present bilaterally.
ABD	Unremarkable.
Back	Urticaria present in upper back, superior to scapulas.
Pelvis	Stable.
Ext	Unremarkable, although the patient says she has tingling in both hands.

Vitals

BP	84/66
P	150, regular
RR	36 shallow
Pupils	PERL 3+ mm
GCS	4+4+6=14
BS	4.1 mmol/l
Pulse oximetry	86%
Skin	Cool, diaphoretic with urticaria

Pain Assessment

O	n/a
P	n/a
Q	n/a
R	n/a
S	n/a
T	n/a

Cardiac Monitor

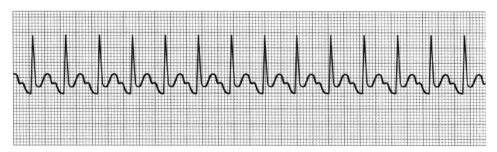

Figure 15.1

Initial Treatment Post Assessment

An assessment should be completed and a complete set of vitals obtained. Oxygen should be administered by a high concentration mask such as a non-rebreather mask. Epinephrine should be administered subcutaneously (SQ) (0.3–0.5 mg). An intravenous should be started and a fluid bolus initiated and titrated to a BP of 100 systolic. If protocol dictates, diphenhydramine should be administered to the patient en route to the hospital. Monitoring of the patient's mentation and respiratory status should be evaluated during transport. Salbutamol may be administered if her wheezing continues post epinephrine administration.

En route, the patient's breathing improves dramatically, her respiratory rate decreases to approximately 20 with a greater tidal volume, and her blood pressure is now 102/78. The patient still complains of a swollen tongue and difficulty swallowing, but the tingling in her hands has now disappeared.

Cardiac Monitor

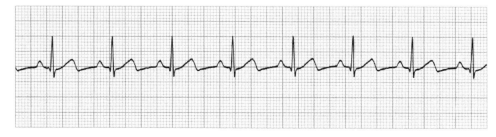

Figure 15.2

Treatment Continued

The IV bolus should be stopped and the IV administered at TKVO. The patient should receive an additional administration of epinephrine SQ. As respiratory distress diminishes, a second salbutamol treatment may not be necessary, but the patient's lung fields should be auscultated for any adventitious sounds.

Differential Diagnosis

- Anaphylaxis.

Test Your Knowledge

1. What ECG is the patient presenting with?
2. Is there a difference between cardiac-administered Xylocaine and Xylocaine administered for freezing?
3. What is the mechanism of action of epinephrine in an anaphylactic patient?
4. What is urticaria, and what causes it?
5. Is the SPO2 of 86 percent significant in the assessment of this patient?
6. With respect to the administration of medication, what are the "Six Rights"?
7. What are typical signs and symptoms of anaphylaxis?

CASE 15.2

You are dispatched at 13:30hrs to 80 Poplar Street, Elliot Lake, Ontario, for a fallen patient. On arrival, you are met by an elderly female and directed to the rear of the house. As you turn the corner to the backyard, you observe an extension ladder on the ground and an elderly male lying next to it. He appears to be awake and is moaning. He is supine and he has an obvious angulated right femur and wrist. It appears as though the patient tried to cushion his fall. His wife tells you that Ralph, who is 65 years old, didn't want to wait for his son Mitch to clean the gutters and went up the ladder himself. She explains that he has a weak heart and shouldn't have been made the attempt. As you approach Ralph, he acknowledges your presence but stays where he has fallen. You are being pestered by wasps as you begin your assessment.

Initial Assessment Findings & Chief Complaint

LOA	Patient appears oriented but confused about the incident.
A	Patent.
B	Slightly laboured, mild wheezing present.
C	Weak radial pulses.
Wet Check	Unremarkable.
CC	Fractured wrist and femur.

History

S	Patient complains of pain in his leg and wrist and says he feels as though he can't catch his breath.
A	ASA.
M	enalapril, Theodur, Cialis, Tylenol 3, Lanoxin, hydrochlorothiazide, Slow-K, ranitidine.
P	Hypertension, CHF, MI at age 57, emphysema, GERD.
L	Breakfast.
E	The patient was on a ladder cleaning gutters and appears to have fallen to the ground. It is unknown whether there was a loss of consciousness. The patient's wife heard a loud noise, came running out to the backyard and found her husband on the ground, then called 911.

Assessment

H/N	Abrasion on right forehead, no JVD, trachea midline, appears to have a rash on the occipital region and right shoulder.
Chest	Unremarkable, equal air entry bilaterally although shallow. Pacemaker scar under left clavicle.
ABD	Soft/non-tender.
Back	Unremarkable, although Ralph complains of pain in the lower lumbar area.
Pelvis	Stable.
Ext	Obvious mid-shaft right femur fracture and right wrist fracture with peripheral pulses.

Vitals

BP	96/70
P	75 regular
RR	20 shallow
Pupils	PERL 3+ mm with cataracts
GCS	4+4+6=14
BS	6.2 mmol/l
Pulse oximetry	92%
Skin	Warm, diaphoretic

Pain Assessment

O	n/a
P	n/a
Q	n/a
R	n/a
S	n/a
T	n/a

Cardiac Monitor

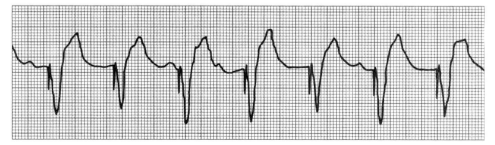

Figure 15.3

Initial Treatment Post Assessment

Because of the mechanism of injury, c-spine alignment should be maintained during assessment of the patient. Post SP02 assessment, oxygen should be administered via a high concentration mask. A blood glucometry should be obtained. Once the assessment is complete, a cervical collar should be applied and the patient secured to a fracture board or scoop stretcher. His wrist should be splinted with a malleable splint to ensure appropriate circulation is present. An IV should be established and a bolus of 20 ml/kg initiated to a systolic pressure of 100. A traction splint should be applied to the patient's right leg en route to the hospital.

During transport, the patient becomes more short of breath and presents with obvious stridor. He says he is having trouble talking and swallowing. His BP has dropped to 78/60, and he is beginning to complain of severe weakness and dizziness. On further assessment of his neck and chest, you notice he is presenting with gross urticaria around three large welts on his shoulder and under the collar you have applied.

Treatment Continued

You now determine that the patient has been stung by some type of insect, possibly one of the wasps at the scene, and is having an allergic reaction. He requires constant monitoring of vitals and ECG interpretation. The patient should receive epinephrine 0.3–0.5 mg SQ as he is now hemodynamically unstable and is presenting with laryngeal edema, dyspnea, and obvious anaphylaxis. The IV bolus should be continued until a systolic pressure of 100 is reached. The patient's fractures should be reassessed en route for the six Ps.

Differential Diagnosis

- Fractured femur and wrist.
- Anaphylaxis.

Test Your Knowledge

1. What are the classifications of the patient's medications?
2. What is your interpretation of the patient's ECG?
3. Why is the patient's blood pressure decreasing?
4. What medication may hinder Ralph's compensatory response by contributing to his falling blood pressure?
5. Your patient has a history of coronary artery disease. Should he be given epinephrine?
6. What effects will epinephrine SQ have on this patient?

Answers
Case 15.1

1. **What ECG is the patient presenting with?**

   The patient is presenting in a sinus tachycardia rhythm progressing to a normal sinus rhythm.

2. **Is there a difference between cardiac-administered Xylocaine and Xylocaine administered for freezing?**

   Xylocaine used during the treatment of cardiac arrest does not contain preservatives, unlike that used for freezing at a dentist's office. The patient may not be allergic to Xylocaine but to the preservative.

3. **What is the mechanism of action of epinephrine in an anaphylactic patient?**

   Epinephrine is a beta-adrenergic drug and, as such, is responsible for heart and lung stimulation. Its alpha-1 properties cause vasoconstriction, leading to a rise in a patient's blood pressure. This is beneficial as it counteracts the vasodilatation of blood vessels caused by anaphylaxis. The beta-2 properties cause bronchodilation, which aids in a respiratory response and reduces wheezing and acute dyspnea caused by allergic reaction.

4. **What is urticaria, and what causes it?**

   Urticaria may present in varying degrees but is characterized by red welts or patches on the body. It is caused by the vasodilation induced by histamines released from mast cells.

5. **Is the SPO2 of 86 percent significant in the assessment of this patient?**

   The SPO2 and combined patient presentation are both significant in the assessment of this patient. The oxygen saturation represents the percentage of oxygen carrying hemoglobin in the blood. Lower pre-hospital oxygen saturation indicates that the patient is not properly exchanging air and is becoming hypoxic.

6. **With respect to the administration of medication, what are the "Six Rights"?**

   The "Six Rights" for medication administration include:
   - Right patient
   - Right time
   - Right medication
   - Right dose
   - Right route
   - Right documentation

7. **What are typical signs and symptoms of anaphylaxis?**

   The typical signs and symptoms of anaphylaxis include:
   - Generalized edema
   - Urticaria
   - Wheezing
   - Stridor
   - Hoarse voice
   - Tachycardia
   - Hypotension/shock
   - Difficulty swallowing
   - Confusion
   - Respiratory distress
   - Nausea/vomiting

Case 15.2

1. *What are the classifications of the patient's medications?*

enalapril (Vasotec)	– ACEI
Theodur (theophylline)	– Bronchodilator
Cialis (tadalafil)	– Erectile dysfunction medication
Tylenol 3 (acetaminophen with codeine)	– Narcotic analgesic
lanoxin (digoxin)	– Cardiac glycoside
hydrochlorothiazide (Hydrodiuril)	– Diuretic
Slow-K (potassium)	– Potassium supplement
ranitidine (Zantac)	– Histamine H2 antagonist (H2 blocker)

2. *What is your interpretation of the patient's ECG?*

   The patient is presenting in a paced rhythm.

3. *Why is the patient's blood pressure decreasing?*

   His blood pressure is decreasing as a result of the vasodilation caused by anaphylaxis.

4. *What medication may hinder Ralph's compensatory response by contributing to his falling blood pressure?*

   Ralph is taking enalapril, an ACE inhibitor. The body's natural response in a crisis with falling blood pressure is to compensate via sympathetic stimulation involving tachycardia and vasoconstriction. Enalapril may be ingested in an attempt to prevent the normal progression of angiotensin I to angiotensin II and the resultant vasoconstriction. However, like enalapril, anaphylaxis also causes vasodilation. The combination of these processes may cause a patient's blood pressure to decrease more rapidly. The sympathetic response will usually overpower the pharmacological response, depending on the amount of drug taken.

5. *Your patient has a history of coronary artery disease. Should he be given epinephrine?*

   Yes, this patient should be given epinephrine, regardless of medical history. Without epinephrine, the patient will succumb to anaphylaxis due to falling blood pressure, bronchoconstriction, and, ultimately, respiratory failure.

6. *What effects will epinephrine SQ have on this patient?*

   The injection of epinephrine SQ (subcutaneously) should cause a sympathetic response and stimulation of alpha and beta receptors. His heart rate should mildly increase and his blood pressure should increase as a result of vasoconstriction. As well, the patient's stridor should diminish and his dyspnea should subside due to bronchodilation and smooth muscle relaxation.

Chapter 16
Gastroenterology

A gastrointestinal emergency is usually the result of an underlying pathological process. Abdominal pain can originate from a variety of causes, each of which can present as somatic or visceral. However, because the organs and contents of the abdomen are confined to a limited space, a differential diagnosis is not always possible. Signs and symptoms, including description of pain, may be an indication of the quadrant in question. Through a thorough assessment, elicited patient history, and incident history, a description of a patient's complaints may aid in determining the underlying problem. The paramedic's priority is to ensure and maintain a patient's ABCs and to facilitate transport to a medical facility, as some gastrointestinal emergencies are surgical cases.

CASE 16.1

You are dispatched shortly after the supper hour to an upstairs apartment at 26 Smith Street, Kitimat, British Columbia, for a patient complaining of abdominal pain. On arrival, you are greeted by a young boy who tells you that his mom is in the living room and is in a lot of pain. Walking through the patient's kitchen, you see many empty boxes marked "Pedro's Pizzeria" as well as other takeout food containers, empty pop cans, potato-chip bags, and a strong smell of cigarette smoke. You surmise that either there was a big party here yesterday, or this family eats takeout regularly. As you approach, you note that the patient, who is curled up in obvious pain in a fetal position on the couch, is relatively obese. The patient tells you that her name is Jean and that she is 40 years old. She says they had pizza for supper and, about 30 minutes later, she started experiencing sharp pain in her stomach just below the ribs. She has vomited twice, the last being bile.

Initial Assessment Findings & Chief Complaint

LOA	Conscious and alert.
A	Patent.
B	Spontaneous and full volume.
C	Strong radial pulses present.
Wet Check	Unremarkable.
CC	Acute abdominal pain for 30 minutes.

History

S	Complaining of epigastric pain, acute in nature.
A	None.
M	Anusol HC, Rolaids, Refluxamine, famotidine, metoclopramide, Gaviscon.
P	Hemorrhoids, GERD, duodenal ulcer, constant heartburn.
L	Supper.
E	The patient had supper and had a sudden onset of upper epigastric pain, the worst she has ever had.

Assessment

H/N	Unremarkable.
Chest	Equal air entry bilaterally.
ABD	Guarding with increased pain in the right upper quadrant on palpation.
Back	Unremarkable.
Pelvis	Stable.
Ext	Equal strength in extremities and good neurological evaluation.

Vitals

BP	128/88
P	75, regular
RR	16 full volume
Pupils	PERL 3+ mm
GCS	4+5+6=15
BS	n/a
Pulse oximetry	98%
Skin	Pale, diaphoretic

Pain Assessment

O	While at rest 30 minutes prior
P	After eating pizza
Q	Sharp
R	Right subcostal margin
S	10/10
T	30 minutes

Cardiac Monitor

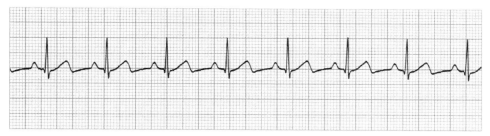

Figure 16.1

Initial Treatment Post Assessment

Initial treatment should include a thorough assessment, including vitals and ECG interpretation. An abdominal assessment should also be performed in order to understand the precursors that may have precipitated the patient's discomfort. Although perfusion and oxygen saturations are adequate, oxygen may be administered via nasal cannula at 28–40%. The patient should be transported in a position of comfort if possible. Care should be taken to position the patient for care of possible emesis. Vitals should be monitored en route to the hospital. There is no rationale to start an intravenous.

Differential Diagnosis

- Cholecystitis.

Test Your Knowledge

1. What is significant about the patient's position when you arrive on scene?
2. What are some of the possible causes of cholecystitis?
3. What are the classifications of the patient's medications?

4. What is the gallbladder's location and function?
5. In a pre-hospital setting, why are analgesics contraindicated?
6. Which narcotic analgesic tends to cause spasm in the cystic duct and is therefore contraindicated in a hospital setting?
7. What sign is evident when pressing on an inflamed gallbladder under the right costal margin?
8. What ECG is the patient presenting with?
9. Could Jean's diet have contributed to her current problem?
10. What exacerbates her condition of GERD?

CASE 16.2

You are dispatched at 13:15hrs to Parkside Junior High School, Altona, Manitoba, for a 15-year-old complaining of abdominal pain and vomiting. On arrival, you are directed to the school's first aid room where you find the patient lying motionless on a bed. The vice principal reports that Tyler came to the office shortly after lunch complaining of pain in his stomach and vomiting. She tells you that he did not eat lunch as he was very nauseated. Tyler is up-to-date with all immunizations, and is not on any medications, and his chart does not reflect any pertinent medical history, although he does have an allergy to peanut butter. You begin talking to Tyler, who tells you that he has not felt well over the previous few days and had a mild stomach ache, which has worsened in the past half-hour. He is febrile and pale.

Initial Assessment Findings & Chief Complaint

LOA	Conscious and alert.
A	Patent.
B	Full volume at 18.
C	Strong radial pulses are present.
Wet Check	Unremarkable.
CC	Abdominal pain.

History

S	Abdominal pain and nausea over the past few days.
A	Peanut butter.
M	EpiPen that Tyler carries with him.
P	None.
L	Breakfast.
E	Tyler complains of nausea and crampy abdominal pain for the past two days, which worsened after lunch and is now sharp.

Assessment

H/N	Unremarkable.
Chest	Equal air entry bilaterally, without adventitious sounds.
ABD	Soft, with visceral tenderness and rebound tenderness in the right lower quadrant.
Back	Unremarkable.
Pelvis	Stable.
Ext	Equal strength and mobility present.

Vitals

BP	118/68
P	75–80 strong/regular
RR	18 full volume
Pupils	PERL 3+ mm
GCS	4+5+6=15
BS	n/a
Pulse oximetry	100%
Skin	Pale, febrile

Pain Assessment

O	Gradual
P	At rest
Q	n/a
R	Peri-umbilicus in right lower quadrant
S	8/10
T	45 minutes (severe)

Cardiac Monitor

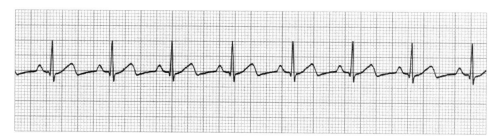

Figure 16.2

Initial Treatment Post Assessment

Initial treatment should include a complete assessment including vitals and ECG interpretation. The patient is perfusing well and has good SPO2, so supplemental oxygen is not required but can be administered based on patient presentation. An incident history should be obtained as well as a thorough abdominal exam, including an assessment of rebound tenderness. An intravenous can be established and run at TKVO and an ACP may administer IV dimenhydrinate if within local protocol. The patient should be transported in a position of comfort, and monitoring of vital signs should continue en route to the hospital.

Differential Diagnosis

- Appendicitis.

Test Your Knowledge

1. What is the physiological function of the appendix?
2. What is the typical presentation of appendicitis?
3. Where is McBurney's point located?
4. What ECG is Tyler presenting with?
5. What may cause the appendix to rupture?
6. Why is appendicitis frequently misdiagnosed?
7. What is a positive psoas sign in the assessment of appendicitis?
8. Why should rebound tenderness only be assessed on Tyler during the initial assessment, and not repeatedly?

CASE 16.3

At 05:30hrs on a Sunday morning, you are dispatched to 12 Fir Lane, Digby, Nova Scotia, for a 55-year-old man vomiting blood. You have been to this rooming house many times before, and prepare by dabbing some Vicks in your nostrils to combat the building's smell of urine and stale alcohol. People who drink XXX or Lysol and need a place to stay nightly, weekly, or monthly commonly reside here. The clientele changes, but the types of calls you receive are the same. Today the door to the apartment is open to reveal your patient, a dishevelled man, sitting on the corner of his bed in his underwear. He has a disproportionately large abdomen for his small frame. He is also pale and diaphoretic. You introduce yourself and he tells you his name is Don.

Initial Assessment Findings & Chief Complaint

LOA	Appears confused.
A	Patent.
B	Shallow but regular.
C	No radial pulses, but carotid pulses are strong.
Wet Check	Yellow urine stains on his underwear.
CC	Vomiting blood.

History

S	Patient is complaining of epigastric pain with nausea and vomiting.
A	None.
M	Antabuse, not taken for two weeks prior, NTG patch (wearing).
P	Stomach disorders, alcoholism, angina.
L	Yesterday, a sandwich at the soup kitchen down the road.
E	Don has been drinking heavily for the past year and admits he is an alcoholic, drinking a 26-oz bottle each day. Over the past few days, he has been drinking continuously. He is unsteady while sitting on his bed. His breath smells of residual alcohol. He tells you that he has been spitting up blood since the previous night and doesn't feel right. He is cold and feels sick.

Assessment

H/N	Unremarkable, no JVD, trachea midline.
Chest	Unremarkable, equal air entry bilaterally to all lobes, with a mild consolidation in the right lower lobe.
ABD	Severely distended with no pain on palpation.
Back	Unremarkable.
Pelvis	Stable.
Ext	Weak, noted muscle wastage, frail.

Vitals

BP	78/58
P	150
RR	20 shallow
Pupils	PERL 5 mm, slow
GCS	4+4+6=14
BS	4.1 mmol/l
Pulse oximetry	88%
Skin	Pale, diaphoretic, slight jaundice present

Pain Assessment

O	Throughout the night
P	At rest
Q	Burning in the chest
R	None
S	6/10
T	Several hours

Cardiac Monitor

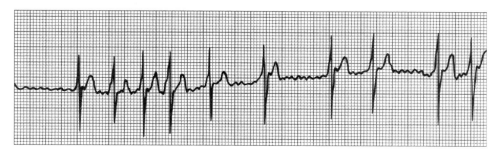

Figure 16.3

Initial Treatment Post Assessment

Initial treatment should include a generalized assessment and a complete set of vitals, including blood glucometry and an ECG interpretation. The patient should be prepared for transport promptly in lieu of his life-threatening condition and presentation. Oxygen should be administered via a high concentration mask at 12–15 lpm. An intravenous should be established and a 20 ml/kg bolus initiated to maintain a systolic pressure of 100. The patient's Nitroglycerin patch should be removed and discarded.

En route to the hospital, the patient vomits copious amounts of blood with clots, overflowing the readied emesis bag. The patient then tells you he feels better. He is grey in colour as you lower him to a supine position. He tells you he just wants to sleep. You are only minutes from the hospital. His vitals are BP 60/40, P 66 (carotid), RR 12, PERL 4+ mm, and SPO2 92%.

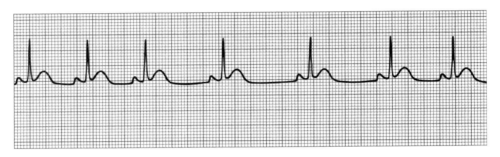

Figure 16.4

Treatment Continued

Monitoring of the patient should be continued, as should oxygen therapy. His airway should be reassessed. The patient should be placed in a semi-prone position and intravenous therapy should continue with the 20 ml/kg bolus. Paramedics should focus on rapid transport to the emergency department.

Differential Diagnosis

- Esophageal varices.

Test Your Knowledge

1. What is esophageal varices?
2. What are the causes of esophageal varices?
3. What ECG is Don presenting in?
4. What are the classifications of Don's medications?
5. What treatment may be initiated upon arrival at the emergency department?
6. How do patients with esophageal varices usually present?

7. Why is the mortality rate high for patients presenting with esophageal varices?
8. What liver disorder may contribute to esophageal varices?

CASE 16.4

At 06:00hrs on a Tuesday morning, you are dispatched to the Delta Prince Edward in Charlottetown, Prince Edward Island, for a 45-year-old male with abdominal pain. On arrival, you are met by the concierge and brought to room 407, where Mr. Tom Sinclair is staying. As you enter, Mr. Sinclair looks uncomfortable, sitting on a wing back chair. He appears pale and is close in colour to the white hotel housecoat he is wearing. He tells you he is in town for three days for a conference and is trying to secure contracts for his company. He says he is under significant stress. He was out entertaining guests yesterday and returned to the hotel around midnight not feeling very well. He drank milk, which seemed to settle his stomach, and went to bed. He awoke with abdominal cramping, nausea, lightheadedness, and black stools.

Initial Assessment Findings & Chief Complaint

LOA	Conscious and alert.
A	Patent.
B	Spontaneous at 16.
C	Weak radial pulses.
Wet Check	Unremarkable.
CC	Nausea, abdominal pain.

History

S	Crampy abdominal pain with nausea and dark, thick diarrhea.
A	None.
M	Ativan, Restoril, Pepcid AC, ibuprofen.
P	Anxiety, heartburn, chronic back pain.
L	20:00hrs last night.
E	Patient came home after a night out and awoke with nausea, dizziness, abdominal pain, and thick black stools.

Assessment

H/N	Unremarkable.
Chest	Equal air entry bilaterally, no adventitious sounds.
ABD	Soft/non-tender on palpation.
Back	Slight back pain.
Pelvis	Stable.
Ext	Unremarkable, equal strength and mobility.

Vitals

BP	98/68
P	150, regular
RR	16 full volume
Pupils	PERL 3+ mm
GCS	4+5+6=15
BS	n/a
Pulse oximetry	96%
Skin	Pale, cool

Pain Assessment

O	This morning
P	Ate last night around 20:00hrs
Q	Crampy
R	None
S	Unable to determine
T	60 minutes

Cardiac Monitor

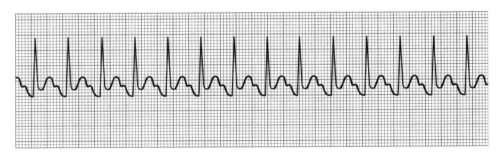

Figure 16.5

Initial Treatment Post Assessment

Initial treatment should include a complete assessment with vitals and an ECG interpretation. The patient should be evaluated for orthostatic hypotension and an intravenous should be established with a 20 ml/kg bolus initiated. The patient should be administered oxygen via a high concentration mask and transported in a position of comfort.

Differential Diagnosis

- Possible duodenal ulcer with upper GI bleed.

Test Your Knowledge

1. Is the time of Mr. Sinclair's last meal significant in your assessment?
2. Is this a possible upper or lower abdominal bleed? Why?
3. What ECG is Mr. Sinclair presenting with?
4. What are the classifications of the patient's medications?
5. What is the presentation of black stools indicative of?
6. What test is performed to determine a loss of circulating volume for which the body is not compensating?

7. What are the major causes of upper and lower GI hemorrhage?
8. Who is more prone to gastric ulcers?

Answers

Case 16.1

1. *What is significant about the patient's position when you arrive on scene?*

   The patient is presenting in a typical position for abdominal injury or discomfort. The fetal position, or knees drawn to the chest, decreases pressure within the abdominal cavity thereby potentially decreasing discomfort.

2. *What are some of the possible causes of cholecystitis?*

   Some of the possible causes of cholecystitis include:

   Gallstones
   Inflammation from bacterial infection
   Burns
   Sepsis
   Diabetes
   Poor or absent blood flow to the gallbladder
   Abnormal metabolism of cholesterol and bile salts

3. *What are the classifications of the patient's medications?*

Anusol HC (hydrocortisone)	– anti-inflammatory cream/suppositories
Rolaids (Rolaids)	– antacid
Refluxamine (Refluxamine)	– soothes smooth muscle in the GI tract
famotidine (Pepcid)	– histamine H2 receptor antagonist
metoclopramide (Maxeran)	– upper GI motility stimulator
Gaviscon (Gaviscon)	– acid neutralizing agent

4. *What is the gallbladder's location and function?*

   The gallbladder is on the undersurface of the liver and stores bile that enters by way of the hepatic duct. When digestion occurs in the stomach, the gallbladder ejects bile into the duodenum.

5. *In a pre-hospital setting, why are analgesics contraindicated?*

   Analgesics are usually contraindicated in a pre-hospital setting as they mask the true presentation of pain and impede assessment and appropriate diagnosis when a patient reaches the emergency department.

6. *Which narcotic analgesic tends to cause spasm in the cystic duct and is therefore contraindicated in a hospital setting?*

   Morphine sulphate.

7. *What sign is evident when pressing on an inflamed gallbladder under the right costal margin?*

   Murphy's sign is the pain caused when an inflamed gallbladder is palpated by pressing under the right costal margin.

8. *What ECG is the patient presenting with?*

   The patient is presenting with a normal sinus rhythm.

9. *Could Jean's diet have contributed to her current problem?*

   Yes, ingestion of fatty foods could trigger a secondary release of bile from the gallbladder.

10. *What exacerbates her condition of GERD?*

The following can contribute to the condition of GERD:

Ingestion of chocolates
Fried foods
Coffee
Smoking
Alcohol

Case 16.2

1. *What is the physiological function of the appendix?*

The appendix is lymphoid in type and has no physiological function.

2. *What is the typical presentation of appendicitis?*

The typical presentation varies from patient to patient, but may start as a visceral peri-umbilical pain or cramp and progress to a more somatic right lower quadrant (RLQ) pain. The patient may complain of nausea and vomiting as well as febrility. Pain in the RLQ may also occur suddenly and without warning.

3. *Where is McBurney's point located?*

McBurney's point is located 4–5 cm anterior to the iliac crest in a direct line with the umbilicus.

4. *What ECG is Tyler presenting with?*

Tyler is presenting with a normal sinus rhythm.

5. *What may cause the appendix to rupture?*

Appendicitis is usually caused by fecal matter obstruction of the appendiceal lumen. Inflammations cause the internal diameter of the lumen to expand, blocking the appendicular artery and causing thrombosis. The appendix then becomes ischemic and necrotic, resulting in the weakening and possible rupture of vessel walls.

6. *Why is appendicitis frequently misdiagnosed?*

Appendicitis is often misdiagnosed because it may present as a visceral pain in the peri-umbilical area. Fever is gradual and may not be evident at the onset of the crampy, diffuse pain. The wide variety and vague nature of symptoms can often mask appendicitis and confound a proper diagnosis.

7. *What is a positive psoas sign in the assessment of appendicitis?*

The psoas sign is an indication of irritation of the iliopsoas group of hip flexors in the abdomen. The test is performed by having a patient lie flat and extend his or her right leg against resistance or drop the leg over the edge of a stretcher or bed. If abdominal pain results, it is a positive psoas sign, since the iliopsoas muscle lies under the appendix when the patient is supine.

8. *Why should rebound tenderness only be assessed on Tyler during the initial assessment, and not repeatedly?*

Continuous rebound tenderness assessments may cause the inflamed appendix to rupture under increased pressure.

Case 16.3

1. *What is esophageal varices?*

Esophageal varices is a swollen vein in the esophagus that often ruptures and hemorrhages. It is usually a result of an increase of portal hypertension. As blood flow to the liver is impeded, blood gets backed up through the left gastric vein and into the esophageal veins. The veins then dilate and outpocket (protrude).

2. *What are the causes of esophageal varices?*

   The typical causes of esophageal varices are the consumption of alcohol or the ingestion of caustic substances such as battery acid or drain cleaner.

3. *What ECG is Don presenting in?*

   The patient is presenting in an atrial fibrillation progressing to a sinus dysrhythmia.

4. *What are the classifications of Don's medications?*

   Antabuse (disulfiram) – produces a highly unpleasant reaction to alcohol
   NTG (nitroglycerin)   – vascular smooth muscle relaxant

5. *What treatment may be initiated upon arrival at the emergency department?*

   If the patient continues to hemorrhage, emergency department treatment may include the insertion of a Sengstaken-Blakemore tube to try to tamponade the rupture.

6. *How do patients with esophageal varices usually present?*

   Patients with esophageal varices may present with painless bleeding and signs of being hemodynamically unstable. As the varices continue to stretch, the patient will progress with more hematemesis, dysphagia, and sensations of burning or tearing pain in the epigastrium.

7. *Why is the mortality rate so high for patients presenting with esophageal varices?*

   The mortality rate is high for patients presenting with esophageal varices because paramedics cannot tamponade the bleeding in a pre-hospital setting.

8. *What liver disorder may contribute to esophageal varices?*

   Cirrhosis of the liver accounts for two-thirds of cases of esophageal varices.

Case 16.4

1. *Is the time of Mr. Sinclair's last meal significant in your assessment?*

   It is important to obtain an estimate of a patient's last oral intake when collecting his or her history. Patients with possible duodenal ulcers usually present with pain at night or early in the morning, when their stomach is empty. Patients with gastric ulcers usually present with pain on a full stomach or just after eating, and not at night.

2. *Is this a possible upper or lower abdominal bleed? Why?*

   This is probably an upper GI bleed because of the presentation of melena—a black, tarry stool. If the blood was frank (i.e., bright red) or the patient presented as hemodynamically stable, these signs would indicate that there was not a significant amount of blood lost.

3. *What ECG is Mr. Sinclair presenting with?*

   The patient is presenting with a sinus tachycardia.

4. *What are the classifications of the patient's medications?*

   Ativan (lorazepam)   – anxiolytic
   Restoril (temazepam) – sedative/hypnotic
   Pepcid AC (famotidine) – H2 receptor antagonist
   ibuprofen (Motrin)   – NSAID

5. *What is the presentation of black stools indicative of?*

   Black, tarry stools are indicative of an upper GI bleed and of partially digested blood which has been in the GI tract for 5–8 hours. Approximately 150 ml/kg of blood must find its way into the GI tract for melena to be recognizable.

6. *What test is performed to determine a loss of circulating volume for which the body is not compensating?*

   The tilt test should be utilized to check for orthostatic hypotension. The body will normally compensate when repositioned from a lying to standing position without significant changes in vitals. A drop in BP of 10 mm Hg or an increase in pulse rate greater than 20 bpm indicates a positive tilt test. The body can usually compensate for approximately 15 percent blood loss without a clinical presentation of hypotension.

7. *What are the major causes of upper and lower GI hemorrhage?*

   The major causes of upper GI hemorrhage include:
   - Esophageal varices
   - Peptic ulcers
   - Gastroenteritis

   The major causes of lower GI hemorrhage include:
   - Crohn's disease
   - Hemorrhoids
   - Colitis
   - Diverticulitis

8. *Who is more prone to gastric ulcers?*

   People over 50 years old and who work in jobs that require physical activity are more prone to gastric ulcers.

Chapter 17
Urology and Nephrology

Renal and urological emergency patients typically present with an acute abdomen; the most common emergencies are renal colic and renal failure. Other issues include urinary tract infections, dysuria, or anuria, particularly in the elderly. While chronic renal failure may be progressive with dialysis as the end result, acute renal failure is routinely caused by trauma. Perfusion is key to the acute failure patient's treatment. Through assessment and a thorough current patient history, a differential diagnosis may be obtained.

CASE 17.1

After picking up a large double-double at your local Tim Horton's at the start of your morning shift, you are dispatched to 14 Jogues Street, Shawinigan, Quebec. As you pull up to the house, you are met by a young man, Jean, who tells you that his 63-year-old father, Maurice Aubin, is confused, and that he has never seen him like this before. Jean says that his dad is usually fine—active and very outgoing. Jean further reports that after being unable to get in touch with his father for the past three days, he decided to check in on him. The patient, Maurice, appears unkempt and is wearing the same clothes he was wearing when his son saw him last.

Initial Assessment Findings & Chief Complaint

LOA	Confused as to time and place.
A	Patent.
B	Shallow at 28.
C	Strong radial pulse, irregular.
Wet Check	Incontinent of urine.
CC	Confused.

History

S	Patient is confused as to time and place and appears to have neglected his day-to-day routines.
A	Codeine.
M	Altace, glyburide, metformin, Lanoxin, Norvasc, HCT, Slow-K.
P	Unable to obtain from patient. The son advises you that Maurice gets his blood cleaned three times a week because his kidneys are not working.
L	CNO.
E	CNO.

Assessment

H/N	JVD present, trachea midline.
Chest	Symmetrical, equal air entry with coarse crackles to the bases bilaterally.
ABD	Soft/non-tender
Back	Unremarkable.
Pelvis	Stable.
Ext	Good range of motion, peripheral edema present in both ankles.

Vitals

BP	156/100
P	100, irregular
RR	28 shallow
Pupils	PERL 3+ mm
GCS	4+4+6=14
BS	3.1 mmol/l
Pulse oximetry	93%
Skin	Cool, damp

Pain Assessment

O	n/a
P	n/a
Q	n/a
R	n/a
S	n/a
T	n/a

Cardiac Monitor

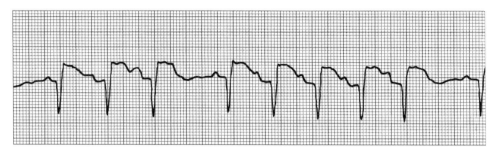

Figure 17.1

Initial Treatment Post Assessment

After an initial assessment, the patient should receive oxygen via a nasal cannula at 4–6 lpm to sustain adequate perfusion and increased saturations. A complete set of vitals and blood glucometry should be obtained as well as an ECG interpretation. An intravenous should be established and run at TKVO, and 1 amp of D50W should be administered. If an IV cannot be initiated, glucagon 1.0 mg should be administered IM or SQ. The patient should be transported in a position of comfort to the emergency department. Constant monitoring should be maintained and blood glucometry repeated if there is no change in the patient's level of awareness.

Differential Diagnosis

- Renal failure with impaired electrolytes.
- Hypoglycemia.

Test Your Knowledge

1. The son advises you that Maurice goes for dialysis three times a week. What types of dialysis are there, and how do they differ?
2. What ECG rhythm is the patient presenting with?
3. What classifications are the patient's medications?

4. What impact does missed dialysis have on a patient's body?
5. What impact does missed dialysis have on the acid-base balance?
6. What is causing the patient's state of confusion?

CASE 17.2

At 07:35hrs, you are dispatched to the North East Arm Hotel in Placentia, Newfoundland, for a 40-year-old female complaining of acute back pain. On arrival at Room 16, the door is opened by a middle-aged man who tells you that his wife, Laura, is in the bathroom. As you approach, the patient exits the bathroom hunched over, pale, and diaphoretic. Laura sits on the bed in obvious pain. Her husband tells you that they are from Ontario and are spending a week touring Newfoundland. Laura has been complaining of intermittent right flank pain for the past few days, since crossing on the ferry. The pain has been relieved with ibuprofen. This morning she was awakened by the pain, however, and it became so unbearable that her husband called the ambulance.

Initial Assessment Findings & Chief Complaint

LOA	Patient is alert and oriented.
A	Patent.
B	Regular and full volume at 16.
C	Strong radial pulses.
Wet Check	Unremarkable.
CC	Right flank pain.

History

S	Sharp intermittent pain in the right flank area radiating to the groin.
A	sulindac.
M	Diamox, allopurinol, Sulcrate, lisinopril, Maxeran.
P	Stomach disorders, hypertension.
L	Breakfast (late): Egg McMuffin.
E	The patient awoke this morning with another episode of severe flank pain. The pain was so severe it made her nauseated to the point she thought she might throw up. She has had three children but has never felt pain like this before.

Assessment

H/N	Unremarkable.
Chest	Air entry equal bilaterally without adventitious sounds present.
ABD	Soft/non-tender on palpation.
Back	No increased pain on palpation.
Pelvis	Stable.
Ext	Unremarkable, no peripheral edema present. Equal strength/mobility.

Vitals

BP	150/94
P	75, regular
RR	16, full volume
Pupils	PERL 3+ mm
GCS	4+5+6=15
BS	n/a
Pulse oximetry	98%
Skin	Pale, diaphoretic

Pain Assessment

O	30 minutes
P	Unprovoked
Q	Sharp
R	To groin
S	10/10, excruciating
T	30 minutes

Cardiac Monitor

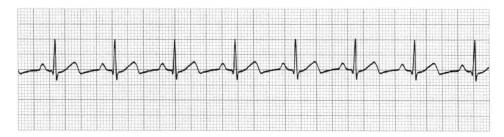

Figure 17.2

Initial Treatment Post Assessment

Initial assessment should include abdominal and pain assessments. The patient should have all vitals and an ECG interpretation completed prior to transport. Although uncomfortable, the patient should be positioned on a stretcher and transported. An intravenous should be initiated and run at TKVO. An ACP may administer narcotic analgesics such as fentanyl or morphine sulphate to make the patient comfortable but not pain-free, as this will make assessment at the emergency department difficult.

Differential Diagnosis

- Renal colic.

Test Your Knowledge

1. What are the typical signs and symptoms of renal colic (calculi)?
2. What causes the acute pain and radiation of pain in renal colic?
3. What are the classifications of the patient's medications?
4. What ECG rhythm is the patient presenting in?
5. How do patients with renal colic differ in presentation from other patients with an acute abdomen?
6. What is the classification of the patient's drug allergy, sulindac?
7. What are the three phases of an acute renal attack?

Answers

Case 17.1

1. *The son advises you that Maurice goes for dialysis three times a week. What types of dialysis are there, and how do they differ?*

   There are two types of dialysis: hemodialysis and peritoneal dialysis.

   Hemodialysis is when a machine containing an artificial filter is attached to a patient via a fistula surgically inserted in the patient's forearm. The patient's blood is filtered through a solution called dialysate and an artificial membrane, then returned to the patient. This process mimics the function of the kidney.

   Peritoneal dialysis uses the abdominal cavity as a semi-permeable membrane and dialysate is infused into the cavity via an indwelling catheter. The fluid is left in the abdomen and drained with impurities via another catheter. This can be completed at home and does not require the patient to go to a hospital for Hemodialysis.

2. *What ECG rhythm is the patient presenting with?*

   The patient is presenting with a second-degree AV block, type 1.

3. *What classifications are the patient's medications?*

Altace (ramapril)	– ACE inhibitor
glyburide (Diabeta)	– Oral hypoglycemic
metformin (Glucophage)	– Oral hypoglycemic
Lanoxin (digoxin)	– Cardiac glycoside
Norvasc (amlodipine)	– Calcium channel blocker
HCT (hydrochlorothiazide)	– Diuretic
Slow-K (potassium)	– Potassium supplement

4. *What impact does missed dialysis have on a patient's body?*

   Without the artificial filtering process that dialysis performs, the body's fluids and electrolytes are affected, which in turn affect all body systems. The cardiovascular system is affected with excessive fluid accumulation leading to hypertension and edema, and can lead to pulmonary edema and respiratory distress. The neurological system is also affected because of an increase in certain electrolytes that affect the nervous system, causing muscle twitching, paresthesia, paralysis, and headaches.

5. *What impact does missed dialysis have on the acid-base balance?*

   Missed dialysis can lead to the accumulation of waste products in the blood as a byproduct of metabolism. These waste products can lead to an accumulation of hydrogen ions, ultimately causing metabolic acidosis.

6. *What is causing the patient's state of confusion?*

   The accumulation of acids (leading to metabolic acidosis) and the state of hypoglycemia could both be causing Maurice's confusion.

Case 17.2

1. *What are the typical signs and symptoms of renal colic (calculi)?*
   The typical signs of renal failure include:

   History focusing on the type and location of pain
   May present as visceral pain in flank on being awoken from sleep
   Increased urinary frequency
   Dysuria
   Painful urination
   Hematuria

Hypertension
Tachycardia

2. *What causes the acute pain and radiation of pain in renal colic?*

   The pain, which usually originates in the upper lateral back (flank) over the costovertebral angle, is a result of the stretching, dilation, and spasm caused by ureteral obstruction. The pain usually radiates inferiorly and anteriorly to the groin.

3. *What are the classifications of the patient's medications?*

Diamox (acetazolamide)	– Carbonic anhydrase inhibitor
allopurinol (Zyloprim)	– Inhibits xanthine oxidase
Sulcrate (sucralfate)	– Ulcer treatment
lisinopril (Zestril)	– ACE Inhibitor
Maxeran (metoclopramide HCl)	– Modifier of upper GI tract motility

4. *What ECG rhythm is the patient presenting in?*

   The patient is presenting in a normal sinus rhythm.

5. *How do patients with renal colic differ in presentation from other patients with an acute abdomen?*

   Patients with renal colic tend to move constantly, trying to find a more comfortable position, while patients with an acute abdomen try to stay motionless.

6. *What is the classification of the patient's drug allergy, sulindac?*

   sulindac (Clinoril)   – Anti-inflammatory, analgesic

7. *What are the three phases of an acute renal colic attack?*

Acute phase:	Onset of pain increasing in intensity
	Usually reaches excruciating pain in as few as 30 minutes
	May reach the maximum pain level 1–2 hours after onset
Constant phase:	Once pain reaches its maximum intensity
	Usually lasts 1–4 hours
	Most patients arrive in the emergency department during this phase
Relief phase:	Pain diminishes quickly
	The patient may fall asleep, particularly if given strong analgesics
	Usually, when the patient wakes up, the pain has disappeared

Chapter 18
Toxicology and Substance Abuse

Toxicological emergencies result from ingestion, inhalation, absorption, or injection of toxic substances. These toxins exert adverse effects on the body's metabolic mechanisms. Many EMS calls are related to the ingestion of toxic substances or substance abuse. Paramedics will encounter patients who have ingested medications or street drugs in an effort to end their life or as an accidental overdose. Judgment should be reserved in these situations; appropriate patient care should always involve an effort to sustain life. Follow-up treatment may be required once a patient has been admitted to hospital. In dealing with toxicological emergencies, the paramedic must recognize the poisoning promptly, perform a thorough assessment, and initiate standard treatment procedures. During assessment, careful attention should be paid to such details as the patient's skin and pupils, as they may help isolate specific toxidromes.

CASE 18.1

At 16:30hrs, you are dispatched to a gym at 480 Linden Avenue, Winnipeg, for a collapsed patient. Upon entering the gym, you are pointed in the direction of a Smith machine. Your patient, a middle-aged male, is sitting propped up against a wall. He appears to have a few friends with him, and is conscious but looks flushed. A friend tells you that Jean-Guy, 30, was lifting weights and had just completed a set when he collapsed. Another friend caught Jean-Guy before he hit the ground, but the patient was out for several minutes. The friend says Jean-Guy has been training hard and taking energy pills. He also says Jean-Guy had two cans of an energy drink before he started his routine.

Initial Assessment Findings & Chief Complaint

LOA	Conscious, confused.
A	Patent.
B	Shallow.
C	Bounding radial pulses.
Wet Check	Unremarkable.
CC	Syncope while weight lifting.

History

S	Confused, syncope.
A	None.
M	Serzone.
P	Depression.
L	Lunch.
E	Jean-Guy was working out and collapsed at the completion of a set, halfway through his workout. His friends could not rouse him for two to three minutes.

Assessment

H/N	No JVD, trachea midline.
Chest	Unremarkable, equal air entry bilaterally. Chest warm and residual diaphoresis present.
ABD	Soft/non-tender.
Back	Unremarkable.
Pelvis	Stable.
Ext	Equally weak grip strength bilaterally. No peripheral edema.

Vitals

BP	200/100
P	250, regular
RR	22
Pupils	PERL 5+ mm
GCS	4+4+6=14
BS	8.4 mmol/l
Pulse oximetry	99%
Skin	hot, flushed,

Pain Assessment

O	n/a
P	n/a
Q	n/a
R	n/a
S	n/a
T	n/a

Cardiac Monitor

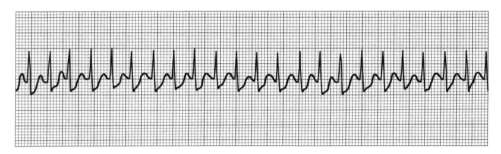

Figure 18.1

Initial Treatment Post Assessment

The patient should be thoroughly assessed and a complete set of vitals obtained, including SPO2 and blood glucometry. The patient should be administered oxygen via a high concentration mask, and cardiac monitoring should be initiated. Jean-Guy should be cooled with cold packs on the groin, neck, and mid-axillary regions. An intravenous should be established and infused at TKVO. The patient should be transported in a position of comfort. An ACP should give supportive care treatment.

While still at the scene, you ask for the patient's belongings. A friend brings Jean-Guy's gym bag and hands you a bottle of ephedra and a bottle of thermogenics. In the bag are two cans of Red Bull as well as a prescription for Serzone.

Treatment Continued

You now have a possible cause for the patient's hypertensive crisis and syncopal episode. The ACP's care should remain supportive: although the patient's presenting rhythm may be treatable, the cause is ingestion, to which rhythm is secondary.

Differential Diagnosis

- Possible overdose of thermogenics, energy drink, and/or ephedra.
- Heat exhaustion.

Test Your Knowledge

1. What is important to determine when you arrive at the gym?
2. What is the coffee equivalence of a can of a typical energy drink?
3. What are some of the common ingredients of energy drinks?
4. What are potential side effects of Ma Huang?
5. What might the results be when combining ephedra and energy drinks?
6. What are common side effects of thermogenics?
7. What ECG is the patient presenting with?
8. What is the classification of the patient's medication?
9. Why should you not take ephedra with MAO inhibitors?

CASE 18.2

You are dispatched at 16:45hrs to 231 Masson Avenue, Oshawa, Ontario, for an unknown problem. The local police have also been dispatched, as has tiered fire department first response. On arrival at the residence, you are directed to the patient by a young woman who tells you that she thinks her sister may have taken too many medications. She reports that Tammy has been depressed for the past month after the death of their mother and was prescribed Surmontil to help her cope. The sister says Tammy had her prescription filled five days earlier, which should last a month as she was prescribed two 25 mg tablets daily. The sister also tells you that Tammy broke up with her boyfriend two days earlier.

Initial Assessment Findings & Chief Complaint

LOA	Patient appears slightly confused and is sitting on the couch when you arrive.
A	Patent.
B	Shallow at approximately 16.
C	Radial pulse is weak but present.
Wet Check	Unremarkable.
CC	Confusion, possible overdose.

History

S	Patient is crying, telling you that she never should have left her boyfriend but that he had been cheating on her for six months. She tells you she is weak and wants to be left alone.
A	penicillin.
M	Surmontil, Xanax, Ortho Tri-cyclen Lo.
P	Mild depression.
L	Lunch.
E	Patient reports that she took the vial of pills approximately one hour earlier. You see four pills on the floor and an empty vial with a label that tells you there were 60 tablets when the prescription was filled.

Assessment

H/N	No JVD, trachea is midline, unremarkable.
Chest	Unremarkable with equal air entry, although shallow.
ABD	Soft/non-tender.
Back	Unremarkable.
Pelvis	Stable.
Ext	Unremarkable, no peripheral edema present.

Vitals

BP	88/64
P	170, regular
RR	16 shallow
Pupils	PERL 5 mm, slow to react
GCS	4+4+6=14
BS	4.3 mmol/l
Pulse oximetry	90%
Skin	Warm, flushed

Pain Assessment

O	n/a
P	n/a
Q	n/a
R	n/a
S	n/a
T	n/a

Cardiac Monitor

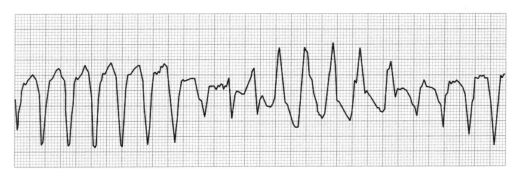

Figure 18.2

Initial Treatment Post Assessment

On arrival, your assessment should attempt to pinpoint the amount of medication taken and when it was ingested. This is important for the ongoing treatment of the patient. Supplemental oxygen should be administered to improve the patient's oxygen saturation. Because of her confused state, a blood glucometry should rule out a hypoglycemic emergency. An IV should be established and a 20ml/kg bolus infused to reach a systolic blood pressure of 100. Because of the patient's cardiac rhythm and confirmed tricyclic ingestion, an ACP should administer sodium bicarbonate 1–2 mlEq/kg. Ongoing assessment of the patient should be continued en route to the hospital, with a focus on respiratory rate and mentation.

En route, the patient's level of consciousness decreases and she eventually becomes unconscious and apneic.

Treatment Continued

An OPA should be inserted and ventilations assisted with a Bag Valve Mask or ATV (Automated Timed Ventilator). Close monitoring of vitals and ECG interpretation should be completed to ensure cardiac output and the absence of cardiac arrest. An ACP should perform oral intubation to secure the patient's airway (use an ETT no. 7–7.5) and confirm placement to eliminate the possibility of aspiration. A fluid bolus should be continued to maintain systolic blood pressure. Sodium bicarbonate administration should continue based on patient presentation.

Differential Diagnosis

- TCA overdose.

Test Your Knowledge

1. What type of depression is Tammy suffering from?
2. What classifications are Tammy's medications?
3. What are the signs of a tricyclic overdose?
4. What other medications produce the same (mainly anticholinergic) toxicological effects as tricyclics?
5. What cardiac rhythm is the patient presenting with?
6. What is the ECG rhythm to which patients may progress when toxic amounts of anticholinergics have been ingested?
7. How many pills do you suspect Tammy has ingested?
8. What is the pharmacology of Surmontil?

CASE 18.3

You are dispatched at 18:00hrs, at the end of a busy day, to 220 Bay Street, Sault Ste. Marie, Ontario, for a patient vomiting blood. On arrival you are met by Jeremy, who leads you to a bathroom where his friend Jay is kneeling in front of the toilet. Jeremy explains that they are a couple and have been together for six months while attending college. This morning he told Jay their relationship was over and that he was going back home to continue schooling there. Jeremy left, then returned around 17:30hrs, when he found Jay in the bathroom. Jay told him he'd taken half of a bottle of ASA at approximately 16:00hrs. Jeremy called 911 immediately. Jay acknowledges your presence and says, "My stomach is killing me."

Initial Assessment Findings & Chief Complaint

LOA	Patient is alert although tired.
A	Patent
B	Tachypneic and slightly laboured.
C	Strong radial pulses present, irregular.
Wet Check	Unremarkable.
CC	Abdominal pain, vomiting blood.

History

S	Patient complaining of acute abdominal pain and vomiting blood tinged vomitus.
A	Tylenol.
M	Tegretol.
P	Epilepsy.
L	Breakfast.
E	Patient admits to taking approximately 100 ASA around 16:00hrs, and had an onset of sharp abdominal pain and vomiting 30 minutes before EMS arrived.

Assessment

H/N	No JVD, trachea midline.
Chest	Unremarkable, equal air entry with shallow respirations and mild crackles bilaterally in the bases.
ABD	Soft, painful on palpation (vague), and guarding.
Back	Unremarkable.
Pelvis	Stable x3.
Ext	Unremarkable, good mobility and distal pulses, capillary refill normal.

Vitals

BP	126/86
P	75, irregular
RR	30
Pupils	PERL 3+ mm
GCS	4+5+6=15
BS	4.1 mmol/l
Pulse oximetry	88%
Skin	Warm, dry

Pain Assessment

O	after ingestion
P	ingestion of ASA
Q	burning
R	none
S	8/10
T	30 minutes

Cardiac Monitor

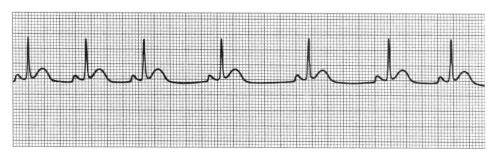

Figure 18.3

Initial Treatment Post Assessment

The patient should be assessed for the amount and time the ASA was ingested. Supplemental oxygen should be administered and cardiac monitoring performed en route to the hospital. The patient should be transported in a position of comfort, preferably in a semi-sitting or sitting position to eliminate the possibility of aspiration if vomiting continues. An IV should be established and run TKVO to eliminate the increased possibility of pulmonary edema. An ACP could administer 1–2 mgEq/kg of sodium bicarbonate to reverse the effects of metabolic acidosis. Blood glucometry should be evaluated throughout transport to treat possible hypoglycemia or DKA.

En route, the patient remains conscious, although his respiratory rate is increasing to close to 40 and he is complaining of ringing in his ears.

Treatment Continued

Supportive care should be continued throughout. No attempt should be made to decrease respirations or administer benzodiazepines, as this would suppress the patient's compensated respiratory rate.

Differential Diagnosis

- ASA overdose.
- Metabolic acidosis with compensatory respiratory alkalosis.

Test Your Knowledge

1. What are the signs of ASA toxicity?
2. What are toxic levels of ASA?
3. What effect does ASA have on the body in relation to Pathophysiology?
4. What ECG is the patient presenting with?
5. The patient is breathing at 40 bpm en route to the hospital. Why would it not be appropriate to try to decrease his respiratory rate?
6. What liniment preparation is equivalent to ASA?
7. Why is the patient presenting with ringing in his ears (tinnitus)?
8. What other medications is the patient taking?

CASE 18.4

You are dispatched at 03:15hrs to an all-night dance club in the lower end of Port Coquitlam, British Columbia, for an unresponsive 18-year-old female. You are met at the front door by a bouncer and the RCMP and led to a crowded dance floor, where the patient lies in her boyfriend Chris's arms. Chris tells you that a group of friends had been dancing all night and that Jodie had begun acting strangely at around 02:30hrs. Soon afterward, Judy slouched in Chris's arms and would not respond to her name. Chris tells you that Judy took some drugs earlier in the night. He is not sure of the type of drug, but he says everyone always does it at this dance club.

Initial Assessment Findings & Chief Complaint

LOA	Patient is confused and unable to answer direct questions.
A	Patent.
B	Regular and full volume.
C	Regular but tachycardic radial pulses.
Wet Check	The patient's shirt is soaked with sweat.
CC	Confused and unable to communicate after a possible drug ingestion and dancing for the past three hours.

History

S	Patient confused and unable to answer questions after having an episode of abnormal behaviour.
A	CNO.
M	CNO.
P	CNO.
L	Supper.
E	The patient was dancing and suddenly had an altered level of consciousness after a change in behaviour. Jodie had been dancing for the previous three hours.

Assessment

H/N	No JVD, trachea midline, unremarkable.
Chest	Unremarkable, equal air entry with no adventitious sounds.
ABD	Soft/non-tender, 4-cm surgical scar on the patient's right lower quadrant.
Back	Unremarkable.
Pelvis	Stable.
Ext	Unremarkable, absent of track marks, capillary refill normal.

Vitals

BP	180/90
P	250
RR	20 regular
Pupils	PERL 6 mm, slow to react
GCS	3+3+5=11
BS	4.6 mmol/l
Pulse oximetry	90%
Skin	Warm, extremely diaphoretic.

Pain Assessment

O	n/a
P	n/a
Q	n/a
R	n/a
S	n/a
T	n/a

Cardiac Monitor

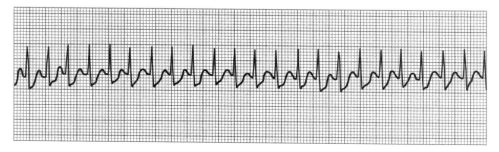

Figure 18.4

Initial Treatment Post Assessment

On arrival, the patient should be moved from the congested dance floor to a quiet area before assessment. Since the patient is awake and protecting her airway, no airway intervention is needed at this time, but an NPA may be required at some point. Oxygen should be administered via a high concentration mask and the patient should be placed in a position of comfort. A thorough assessment should be performed, and the medic should look for track marks. Because of the patient's altered level of consciousness, a blood glucometry should be completed. Cardiac monitoring should occur throughout, and an intravenous should be established and run TKVO. The patient appears febrile, so cold packs should be placed in the axillary and groin regions as well as behind the patient's head in an attempt to cool her.

En route to the hospital, the patient remains warm to touch and appears to become more lethargic. There is no change in her ECG.

Treatment Continued

Monitoring and cooling of the patient is paramount en route to the hospital. An airway adjunct, such as an NPA, should be utilized to help maintain airway patency.

Differential Diagnosis

- 3, 4 Methylenedioxymethamphetamine (MDMA) overdose.

Test Your Knowledge

1. Why is a blood glucometry beneficial with this patient?
2. What is the significance of the patient's skin being very warm to the touch?
3. What is your interpretation of the patient's ECG?
4. What is the mechanism of action of MDMA?
5. What are street names for MDMA?
6. What are the signs and symptoms of an MDMA overdose?
7. What leads to cardiac arrest in an MDMA overdose?
8. What type of surgery would leave a scar on the right lower quadrant?

CASE 18.5

It is 12:30hrs on a warm July day when you are dispatched to 1445 Paquette Avenue, Fort Saskatchewan, for a 65-year-old female who has had a syncopal episode. On arrival, you observe a woman sitting up against her kitchen cupboards. She is conscious and acknowledges your entry, apologetically saying, "I'm sorry to bother you, but I'm not sure what happened." She reports that her leg hurts, and you notice a cane beside her. Her daughter tells you that her mom was sitting at the table when she went downstairs to let the dog in and heard a thud.

Initial Assessment Findings & Chief Complaint

LOA	Patient appears to be distant but focuses on you.
A	Patent.
B	Regular and shallow.
C	Barely palpable radial pulses. Femoral pulse present.
Wet Check	Unremarkable.
CC	Syncopal episode.

History

S	Patient complains of feeling dizzy and having blurred vision.
A	None.
M	Vasotec, atenolol, NTG, Duragesic patches, Tylenol 3.
P	Hypertension, MI at age 60, hip replacement (left) one month prior, osteoarthritis.
L	Breakfast (porridge, prune juice).
E	The patient had just sat down for lunch when she became weak and collapsed to the floor. She tells you she remembers feeling hot, and then waking up on the floor. She tells you her left hip has been extremely sore and she has been applying patches and taking two Tylenol 3 every two hours since the previous day. She says the pain will not go away.

Assessment

H/N	Unremarkable.
Chest	Unremarkable, with equal air entry bilaterally.
ABD	Soft/non-tender.
Back	Unremarkable.
Pelvis	Stable.
Ext	Equal strength/mobility in all extremities. Mild peripheral edema present in both ankles. Scars on left hip (healed well). Capillary refill is delayed and peripheral pulses are absent. A Duragesic patch is present on left upper arm.

Vitals

BP	70/48
P	30, regular
RR	10
Pupils	Pinpoint, non-reactive
GCS	4+5+5=14
BS	4.8 mmol/l
Pulse oximetry	86%
Skin	Pale, diaphoretic

Pain Assessment

O	n/a
P	n/a
Q	n/a
R	n/a
S	n/a
T	n/a

Cardiac Monitor

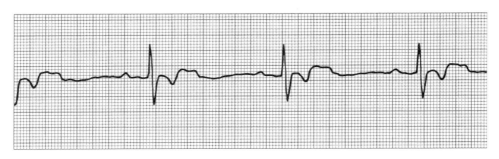

Figure 18.5

Initial Treatment Post Assessment

The patient should be given supplemental oxygen via a high concentration mask to aid in her reduced oxygen saturation. Cardiac monitoring should continue throughout the call. Because of the mechanism of injury and age of the patient, c-spine immobilization should be completed. The patient should be moved to a stretcher after application of a collar and immobilization on a board. Blood glucometry should also be performed to rule out other possible causes of the patient's syncope. An IV should be initiated and a bolus of 20 ml/kg administered to maintain a blood pressure of 100 systolic. An ACP should administer 0.4–0.8 mg naloxone to reverse possible narcotic effects, and the Duragesic patch should be removed.

En route to the hospital, the patient remains weak. Her vitals have improved to BP 104/68, P 58 in a sinus bradycardia, and RR 14. The patient tells you she is tired and wants to go home.

Treatment Continued

The IV bolus should be discontinued and run at TKVO. Continuous monitoring of the patient, including vitals every five minutes, is important. A repeat blood glucometry may be warranted if her level of mentation changes again.

Differential Diagnosis

- Narcotic overdose (unintentional).

Test Your Knowledge

1. What ECG rhythm is the patient presenting in?
2. Why would you settle this patient in a supine position?
3. What are the classifications of medications that the patient is taking?
4. What are the typical signs and symptoms of a narcotic overdose?
5. Why is this patient exhibiting signs and symptoms of a narcotic overdose?
6. Why is it important to remove the Duragesic patch?
7. Is this patient suicidal?

CASE 18.6

You are working a night shift when you are dispatched at 03:30hrs to 40 Gerrard Street, Toronto, for a possible unconscious patient. The city streets are deserted except for the odd passerby. You are only blocks from the call location, so your response time is minimal. As you arrive, you see a city police officer standing over a young man who looks about 19 years old. The police officer reports that the young man has no ID and, from what he can figure, was climbing a statue and fell some six metres to the ground. As you approach the supine patient, you notice he is unkempt. His eyes are open but he doesn't respond to your introduction.

Initial Assessment Findings & Chief Complaint

LOA	Patient opens his eyes to painful stimuli and appears confused when you ask a question.
A	Appears patent.
B	Slow and shallow at approximately 10.
C	Strong radial pulse.
Wet Check	Incontinent of urine and feces, blood behind the patient's head.
CC	Fall, unknown trauma.

History

S	Patient appears to have fallen approximately six metres to the ground.
A	CNO.
M	Ritalin, found in the patient's pocket.
P	CNO.
L	CNO, but there is a McDonald's bag with a half-eaten hamburger lying beside the patient.
E	Possibly climbing a statue and fell approximately six metres, though this was not witnessed.

Assessment

H/N	No JVD, trachea midline, approximately 8-cm laceration on the left temporal lobe of the skull. Bleeding is minimal at this time, but approximately 300 ml are on the ground under the patient.
Chest	Unremarkable, equal air entry.
ABD	Soft/non-tender.
Back	Abrasions on back and a possible dislocation of the left shoulder.
Pelvis	Stable x3.
Ext	Minor abrasions noted on both hands and arms. Track marks noted on both antecubital fossa regions. A capped syringe is found in the patient's right front pants pocket.

Vitals

BP	190/150
P	170
RR	10
Pupils	7 mm, slow to react
GCS	2+4+5=11
BS	3.1 mmol/l
Pulse oximetry	90%
Skin	Warm, diaphoretic

Pain Assessment

O	n/a
P	n/a
Q	n/a
R	n/a
S	n/a
T	n/a

Cardiac Monitor

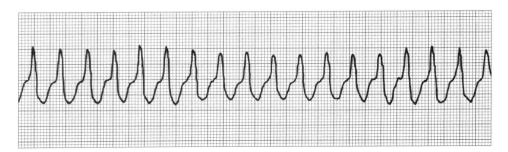

Figure 18.6

Initial Treatment Post Assessment

Because of the possible mechanism of injury, c-spine support should be maintained during your initial assessment. It is important to note that although the patient is not responding well to your questions, his airway is patent and being maintained. Oxygen saturations are low, so the patient should be administered high concentration oxygen. The patient should be completely immobilized on a fracture board or scoop stretcher after a collar has been applied, and an IV should be established and run at TKVO.

As you finish c-spine immobilization post assessment, the patient has a tonic-clonic seizure lasting approximately 30 seconds. After 30 seconds the patient appears post-ictal, and responds only to painful stimuli with decorticate movement. His respiratory rate is still approximately 10 bpm and he has a strong radial pulse.

Treatment Continued

Post-seizure, you reassess your patient's airway, respiratory, and circulatory status, and, now that time allows, conduct a blood glucometry. As his glucometry is low, the patient should receive 25 mg D50W (1 amp) via IV or Glucagon 1.0 mg IM/SQ. His head wound should be dressed as it is still oozing blood. In the absence of a gag reflex, the patient should tolerate an OPA and ventilations should be assisted en route to the hospital. An ACP should perform endotracheal intubation in the absence of a gag reflex. Nasal intubation should be avoided because of the possible head injury. Blood glucometry should be repeated en route.

Blood glucometry is repeated on the way to the hospital and is found to be 8.7 mmol/l.

Differential Diagnosis

- Methamphetamine overdose.

Test Your Knowledge

1. What are the common signs of drug abuse found in this patient? What are other signs?
2. What is Ritalin, and why might the patient be taking it?
3. What may be the drug of choice of this patient, based on his physical presentation?
4. What are the typical signs and symptoms of this classification of street drug?
5. What ECG rhythm is the patient presenting in?
6. What is the definitive treatment for methamphetamine overdose?
7. Why did the patient have a seizure?
8. What are other signs and symptoms relating to methamphetamine intoxication?

CASE 18.7

You are dispatched at 14:50hrs to 17 Everglen Crescent, Souris, Quebec, for a possible attempted suicide. Dispatch advises that the patient is a 17-year-old male found in a garage with a vehicle engine running. Friends on scene have removed him from the car and have begun to perform rescue breathing. As you pull into the driveway, you notice a male and female kneeling beside the patient. One of the teens is providing artificial resuscitation to the patient. You notice the patient appears lifeless and flushed. The female friend tells you they popped in to see Tim after school and noticed exhaust coming from the garage. When they opened the garage door, they saw the car parked and Tim slouched in the front seat. They shut off the engine and took him outside.

Initial Assessment Findings & Chief Complaint

LOA	Unresponsive to verbal or painful stimuli.
A	Patent.
B	Absent.
C	Weak radial pulse.
Wet Check	Unremarkable.
CC	Unconscious—possible carbon monoxide poisoning.

History

S	Patient found unconscious in a car parked in a garage with its engine running.
A	CNO.
M	CNO.
P	Diabetes (MedicAlert necklace).
L	Friend states patient had lunch at school.
E	According to the friend, the patient left school at the same time as him, 14:30hrs, and was heading straight home. The friend tells you that Tim wasn't himself today and seemed preoccupied.

Assessment

H/N	Face flushed, trachea midline, no JVD.
Chest	Unremarkable.
ABD	Unremarkable.
Back	Unremarkable.
Pelvis	Stable x3.
Ext	Unremarkable, weak palpable radial pulse, capillary refill delayed.

Vitals

BP	102/66
P	120, regular
RR	4 shallow
Pupils	PERL 6 mm, slow to react
GCS	1+1+1=3
BS	4.8 mmol/l
Pulse oximetry	84%
Skin	Warm, flushed

Pain Assessment

O	n/a
P	n/a
Q	n/a
R	n/a
S	n/a
T	n/a

Cardiac Monitor

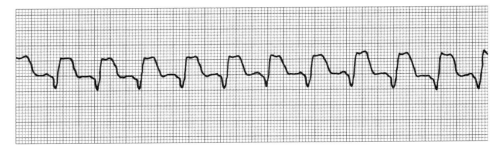

Figure 18.7

Initial Treatment Post Assessment

The patient should be assessed for circulation and other possible injuries. An airway adjunct, such as an OPA, should be inserted, and hyperoxygenation should continue with a BVM. An ACP should initiate endotracheal intubation because of the patient's low GCS and spontaneous respirations of four. As the patient is a medium-size adult, an ETT no. 8.0 should suffice, with confirmation of tube placement and approximately 22–23 cm at the teeth. Cardiac monitoring should be initiated. Routine blood glucometry should be performed and an IV initiated and run at TKVO for possible interventions throughout the call.

Just prior to leaving, the friend notices empty prescription vials in the garbage can in the garage. He runs them over to you before you depart. The first name on the vial does not match the patient's, but the surname is the same. The friend tells you that they are Tim's mother's medications: Luvox, Benadryl, Tylenol, and atenolol.

Treatment Continued

Ventilation should be continued and a ventilator could be utilized to provide more accurate oxygenation and tidal volume levels. Rapid transport to a medical facility should be initiated, where there may be access to a hyperbaric chamber. The patient's ECG should be monitored en route to watch for widening of the QRS. Should it widen, sodium bicarbonate may be administered (2 mEq/kg) to decrease the width of the QRS complex and possibly prevent further deterioration to a lethal rhythm. The patient's blood pressure and other vitals should be monitored, and if his BP falls to below 100 P, fluid boluses should be initiated.

Differential Diagnosis

- Carbon monoxide poisoning.
- Anticholinergic overdose (Benadryl).
- Other overdose of medications.

Test Your Knowledge

1. The friend finds empty medication vials of Luvox, Benadryl, Tylenol, and atenolol in the garage garbage can. What are the classifications of these medications?
2. What ECG is the patient presenting with?
3. What are typical signs and symptoms of a carbon monoxide overdose?
4. What impact does CO poisoning have on a patient's SPO2?
5. Based on the patient's presentation, he has possibly ingested medications in an attempt to take his life. Which medications are directly related to his current state?
6. What mnemonic is used to remember the signs and symptoms of an anticholinergic overdose?

CASE 18.8

On a Sunday morning at approximately 02:30hrs, you are dispatched for an unresponsive patient at the Space Odyssey on Howe Street, Vancouver. On arrival you are greeted by a bouncer, who tells you that a guy is acting as if he is in a trance, freaking everyone out and hugging a chair. The bouncers can't get him out of the bar. The bouncer brings you to a few of the patient's friends, who tell you that Michael smoked some Magic Mint about 10 minutes before coming to the bar. He also had about six bottles of Vex at another bar down the road. As you approach, you see Michael clinging to a bar stool, looking dazed.

Initial Assessment Findings & Chief Complaint

LOA	Conscious, but dazed.
A	Patent.
B	Shallow.
C	Strong radial.
Wet Check	Unremarkable.
CC	Patient is in a trance-like presentation.

History

S	Patient is staring into space.
A	CNO.
M	CNO.
P	CNO.
L	Finger food at the previous bar.
E	The patient's friend tells you that Michael had a few drinks earlier and smoked Salvia before entering the bar. He was okay for a while but then sat on the floor staring into space. He then began clinging to a bar stool and would not let go. The bouncers tried to throw him out but didn't want to make a scene, so they called 911.

Assessment

H/N	No JVD, trachea midline.
Chest	Unremarkable with equal air entry bilaterally.
ABD	Soft/non-tender.
Back	Unremarkable.
Pelvis	Stable.
Ext	Equal strength and mobility.

Vitals

BP	128/88
P	70, irregular
RR	16
Pupils	PERL 4+ mm
GCS	4+4+5=13
BS	4.8 mmol/l
Pulse oximetry	98%
Skin	Warm, diaphoretic

Pain Assessment

O	n/a
P	n/a
Q	n/a
R	n/a
S	n/a
T	n/a

Cardiac Monitor

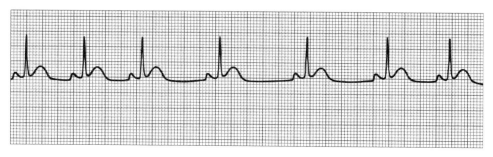

Figure 18.8

Initial Treatment Post Assessment

The patient should be approached slowly, and a complete assessment performed. A baseline set of vitals should be taken, including SPO2 and blood glucometry. Oxygen should be administered and the patient transported to the emergency department. Supportive care should be implemented and vitals reassessed en route. No interventions are required at this time.

En route, the patient becomes more alert and has minimal recollection of the incident at the bar. He remembers being with his friends at the first bar and smoking Salvia. He is cooperative and calm for the remainder of the transport.

Differential Diagnosis

- Ingestion of salvia divinorum.

Test Your Knowledge

1. What are other common names of salvia divinorum?
2. What is Salvia?
3. How is Salvia usually ingested?

4. What is the timeline from ingestion to peak effect to a return to a pre-ingestion state?
5. What are some of the effects of ingesting Salvia?
6. What ECG is the patient presenting with?
7. How do people usually feel after the drug has worn off?

Answers
Case 18.1

1. *What is important to determine when you arrive at the gym?*
   On arrival, it is important to determine the mechanism of injury and the possibility of spinal injury from the fall. It is also imperative to determine if Jean-Guy is on any medications or athletic supplements that may have contributed to the incident or may complicate treatment.
2. *What is the coffee equivalence of a can of a typical energy drink?*
   One can of a typical energy drink containing guarana is equivalent to two cups of coffee.
3. *What are some of the common ingredients of energy drinks?*
   Some of the common ingredients of energy drinks include

Guarana:	From the Paullinia cupana plant
	Source of caffeine
	Stimulant
Taurine:	Amino acid
	Plays a role in fat emulsification
Pyrodoxin:	Member of the B-complex family
	Used in the breakdown of proteins, fats, and carbohydrates for energy

4. *What are potential side effects of Ma Huang?*
   Ma Huang or ephedra—an active ingredient in Jean-Guy's ephedra drink—may cause the following:

   Hypertension
   Tachycardia
   Heart palpitations
   Irritability
   Headache

5. *What might the results be when combining ephedra and energy drinks?*
   Ma Huang, or ephedra, is an active alpha- and beta-andrenergic stimulant that increases heart rate, blood pressure, and cardiac output. Guarana, an active ingredient in energy drinks, can also cause an increase in cardiac output. Both substances are stimulants which lead to overstimulation of the conduction system and the possibility of dysrhythmias.
6. *What are common side effects of thermogenics?*
   Common side effects of thermogenics include:

   Increased metabolism
   Elevated temperature

7. *What ECG is the patient presenting with?*
   The patient is presenting with a supraventricular tachycardia.
8. *What is the classification of the patient's medication?*
   Serzone (nefazodone)   – MAO inhibitor
9. *Why should you not take ephedra with MAO inhibitors?*
   Ephedra and MAO inhibitors should not be taken together as they increase the risk of a hypertensive crisis.

Case 18.2

1. *What type of depression is Tammy suffering from?*
   Tammy is suffering from an exogenous depression brought on by the death of her mother and her recent relationship breakup.

2. *What classifications are Tammy's medications?*

   Surmontil (trimipramine maleate) — Antidepressant
   Xanax (alprazolam) — Anxiolytic
   Ortho Tri-cyclen Lo (norgestimate & ethinyl estradiol) — Birth control pill

3. *What are the signs of a tricyclic overdose?*

   Warm, flushed, dry skin
   Mydriasis
   Tachycardia
   Hypotension
   Dysrhythmias, including Torsade de Pointes, widened QRS segment, or heart block
   Depressed respiratory system
   Seizures

4. *What other medications produce the same (mainly anticholinergic) toxicological effects?*
   The following classifications produce the same effects as TCA overdoses: muscle relaxants, antiparkinson drugs, anti-emetic drugs, some plants, anti-psychotics, and antihistamines.

5. *What cardiac rhythm is the patient presenting with?*
   The patient is presenting in Torsade de Pointes (TdP).

6. *What is the ECG rhythm to which patients may progress when toxic amounts of anticholinergics have been ingested?*
   Patients usually progress from sinus tachycardia to a cardiac dysrhythmia such as Torsade de Pointes or ventricular tachycardia. The progression of the rhythm includes a possible prolonged PR interval, prolonged QT interval, and PVCs. Many patients with a TCA overdose will have a widening of the QRS that may be a precursor to VT or TdP.

7. *How many pills do you suspect Tammy has ingested?*
   The original prescription was filled five days earlier when she received 60 25-mg tablets from a pharmacist. At two pills per day, she should have taken 10 tablets, leaving her with 50. You found four tablets on the floor; therefore, there are 46 tablets missing (1150 mg).

8. *What is the pharmacology of Surmontil?*
   Trimipramine is a TCA antidepressant with sedative properties. It has anticholinergic properties and potentiates the sympathetic response by blocking the reuptake of norepinephrine released by presynaptic neurons. It also has a quinidine-like effect on the heart.

Case 18.3

1. *What are the signs of ASA toxicity?*
   The signs of ASA toxicity are:

   Change in rate and depth of respiration (hyperventilating)
   Increased body temperature
   Nausea
   Abdominal pain
   Blood-tinged vomitus
   Lethargy
   Tinnitus

Confusion
Seizures
Noncardiogenic pulmonary edema

2. *What are toxic levels of ASA?*
   The therapeutic dose of ASA is 15 mg/kg; the toxic dose is 150 mg/kg.

3. *What effect does ASA have on the body in relation to Pathophysiology?*
   Uncouples oxidative phosphorylation
   Decreased ATP
   Increased catabolism and oxidation
   Increased heat release
   Increased oxygen consumption
   Increased CO_2 production
   Increased gluconeogenesis
   Lipid breakdown, ketosis
   Direct stimulation of the respiratory centre (respiratory alkalosis)
   Anaerobic metabolism
   Hyperthermia

4. *What ECG is the patient presenting with?*
   The patient is presenting with a sinus dysrhythmia.

5. *The patient is breathing at 40 bpm en route to the hospital. Why would it not be appropriate to try to decrease his respiratory rate?*
   The increase in respiratory rate is a direct compensation for metabolic acidosis. Any decrease in the respiratory rate, using benzodiazepines, for example, would result in acute acidosis and death.

6. *What liniment preparation is equivalent to ASA?*
   Oil of Wintergreen has similar properties to ASA, and a teaspoon of this liniment is equivalent to 20 ASA tablets.

7. *Why is the patient presenting with ringing in his ears (tinnitus)?*
   Tinnitus is a sign that a significant amount of ASA has gone into the central nervous system.

8. *What other medications is the patient taking?*
   Tegretol (carbamazepine) – Anticonvulsant, antimanic

Case 18.4

1. *Why is a blood glucometry beneficial with this patient?*
   Blood glucometry is an important diagnostic tool for Judy as she has an altered level of consciousness, and you must therefore rule out any hypo/hyperglycemic emergencies.

2. *What is the significance of the patient's skin being very warm to the touch?*
   The patient may have an elevated temperature, presenting with warm or hot skin, because of hyperthermia caused by the ingestion of MDMA.

3. *What is your interpretation of the patient's ECG?*
   The patient is presenting in a supraventricular tachycardia (SVT).

4. *What is the mechanism of action of MDMA?*
   The mechanism of action of MDMA is:
   MDMA is taken orally and dissolved in the stomach
   Some molecules are absorbed, but most enter the intestine with changed polarity (+H)
   Hydrogen (H) ions are released and the drug diffuses through the capillaries
   Some of the drug is metabolized at the liver, but the majority travels to the heart and lungs

MDMA is then carried to organs and the brain
MDMA crosses the brain barrier
Substantial amounts of the drug enter the brain

5. *What are street names for MDMA?*
Street names for MDMA are ecstasy, the love drug, cloud nine, Adam, and ultimate xphoria.

6. *What are the signs and symptoms of an MDMA overdose?*
The signs and symptoms of an MDMA overdose are:

Increased thirst
Altered level of consciousness
Tachycardia
Hyperventilation
Elevated T-waves
Cardiac arrhythmias
Warm or hot skin

7. *What leads to cardiac arrest in an MDMA overdose?*
Cardiac arrest and death due to an MDMA overdose can be caused by:

Dehydration
Hyperthermia
Rhabdomyolysis
Acute renal failure
Tachycardia
Arrhythmias
Convulsions
Dilutional hyponatremia (water intoxication)

8. *What type of surgery would leave a scar on the right lower quadrant?*
The patient may have had an appendectomy.

Case 18.5

1. *What ECG rhythm is the patient presenting in?*
The patient is presenting in a second-degree AV block, type 2.

2. *Why would you settle this patient in a supine position?*
The patient should be placed in a supine position because of her hypotensive state. She fell to the floor from a sitting position prior to the initiation of 911. By having her remain supine on your stretcher, venous return will be increased and, hopefully, will assist in raising her blood pressure.

3. *What are the classifications of medications that the patient is taking?*

Vasotec (enalapril)	– ACE inhibitor
atenolol (Lopressor)	– Beta blocker
NTG (nitroglycerine)	– Vasodilator
Duragesic (fentanyl)	– Narcotic analgesic
Tylenol 3 (Acetaminophen with codeine 30 mg)	– Narcotic analgesic

4. *What are the typical signs and symptoms of a narcotic overdose?*
The typical signs and symptoms of a narcotic overdose include:

Miosis
Diaphoresis
Hypotension
Bradycardia

Confusion
Nausea and vomiting
Respiratory depression
Coma
Death

5. *Why is this patient exhibiting signs and symptoms of a narcotic overdose?*
   This patient is exhibiting signs and symptoms of a narcotic overdose because she is wearing a Duragesic patch (a narcotic) while taking two Tylenol 3 (30 mg codeine each) pills every two hours. The standard dosage of Tylenol 3 is 1–2 tablets every 4–6 hours when required. The patient has been taking three times the normally prescribed dosage and is still wearing a Duragesic patch.

6. *Why is it important to remove the Duragesic patch?*
   It is important to remove the Duragesic patch because as long as it remains on the patient's skin, the narcotic medication is being topically absorbed. Removal of the patch will stop the absorption process. It is important to utilize appropriate PPE, such as gloves, to remove the patch in order to eliminate any possibility of Duragesic being absorbed into the paramedic's skin.

7. *Is this patient suicidal?*
   No, this patient is not suicidal. In the treatment of the acute pain in her hip and osteoarthritis, she has ingested too many Tylenol 3, particularly given her Duragesic patch application. The patient's moderate confusion may also have compounded the situation, since she may have been forgetful as to when she took her medications. She may have repeated them, thinking she had not taken any because she was still experiencing pain.

Case 18.6

1. *What are the common signs of drug abuse in this patient? What are other signs?*
   The most obvious signs and symptoms of drug abuse in this patient are track marks on both forearms and the syringe found in his pocket.

2. *What is Ritalin and why might the patient be taking it?*
   Ritalin (methylphenidate hydrochloride) – Mild central nervous system stimulant
   The patient may be taking this medication for attention deficit disorder or other hyperactive disorders.

3. *What may be the drug of choice of this patient based on his physical presentation?*
   Based on the patient's presentation, the patient uses and has possibly overdosed on a methamphetamine.

4. *What are the typical signs and symptoms of this classification of street drug?*
   Methamphetamine is a sympathomimetic; in other words, it stimulates the sympathetic nervous system. The typical signs and symptoms of a methamphetamine overdose are:

   Profuse sweating
   Rapid breathing
   Increased heart rate
   Mydriasis
   Extreme blood pressure increase
   Unconsciousness

5. *What ECG rhythm is the patient presenting in?*
   The patient is presenting in a ventricular tachycardia.

6. *What is the definitive treatment for methamphetamine overdose?*
   The proper treatment for methamphetamine is supportive care. Once methamphetamine is in the patient's bloodstream it cannot be removed except through the body's normal metabolism.

Chapter 18 Toxicology and Substance Abuse

Overdoses must be treated symptomatically by lowering the body temperature with a cooling blanket and using pharmacology to lower the patient's heart rate and blood pressure (e.g., through the use of beta blockers and calcium channel blockers)

7. **Why did the patient have a seizure?**
   The patient may have had a seizure for several reasons, including hypoglycemia, hyperthermia, or a possible head injury.

8. **What are other signs and symptoms relating to methamphetamine intoxication?**
   Other signs and symptoms of methamphetamine intoxication are:

   Pulmonary edema (non-cardiogenic)
   Hypoglycemia
   Intracerebral hemorrhage
   Hyperthermia
   Hypertension
   Delirium
   Hyperactivity

Case 18.7

1. **The friend finds empty medication vials of Luvox, Benadryl, Tylenol, and atenolol in the garage can. What are the classifications of these medications?**

Luvox (fluvoxamine)	– Selective serotonin reuptake inhibitor (SSRI)
Benadryl (diphenhydramine)	– Antihistamine
Tylenol (acetaminophen)	– Analgesic, anti-pyretic
Atenolol (Tenormin)	– Beta blocker

2. **What ECG is the patient presenting with?**
   The patient is presenting in an accelerated junctional rhythm.

3. **What are typical signs and symptoms of a carbon monoxide overdose?**
   The typical signs and symptoms of CO poisoning are:

   Tachycardia
   Hypertension or hypotension
   Possible tachypnea
   Pallor, although cherry red skin is a late sign
   Noncardiogenic pulmonary edema
   Lethargy
   Coma
   Respiratory arrest

4. **What impact does CO poisoning have on a patient's SPO2 reading?**
   The SPO2 reading may be normal (98–100%), even though the patient may have severe CO poisoning. A traditional pulse oximeter is incapable of distinguishing dyshemoglobins. Pulse oximeters will display an oxygen saturation that is approximately equal to the percentage of hemoglobin combined with oxygen, plus the percentage of hemoglobin combined with CO. If 25 percent of a patient's hemoglobin is saturated with CO and has a true oxygen saturation of 70 percent, a traditional pulse oximeter will display an SPO2 of about 95 percent. Traditional pulse oximetry is of no value in patient assessment in the presence of high concentrations of COHb (carboxyhemoglobin).

5. **Based on the patient's presentation, he has possibly ingested medications in an attempt to take his life. Which medications are directly related to his current state?**
   The patient's current state may be caused by a combination of CO poisoning and the ingestion of medications found at the scene. Because of the tachycardia, mydriasis, and warm and dry skin, it

appears that the patient is experiencing an anti-cholinergic response. Benadryl, although an antihistamine, has anti-cholinergic properties similar to a tricyclic overdose. The anti-cholinergic effects include:

Blockage of norepinephrine
Sodium channel blocker
Peripheral alpha blocker
Inhibition of SNS reflexes
Increased refractory period
Raise in stimulation threshold with decrease in cardiac conduction velocity
Possible widening of the QRS

6. *What mnemonic is used to remember the signs and symptoms of an anti-cholinergic overdose?*

Red as a beet
Hot as a hare
Mad as a hatter
Blind as a bat
Dry as a bone

Case 18.8

1. *What are other common names of salvia divinorum?*
Other common names of salvia divinorum (Salvia) include:

Diviner's sage
Sally D
Magic Mint

2. *What is Salvia?*
Salvia is a powerful psychoactive plant from the mint and sage family. It is considered to be one of the most potent naturally-occurring psychoactive compounds. Salvia has no actions on the serotonin receptors.

3. *How is Salvia usually ingested?*
Salvia is usually eaten (i.e., the leaves are cut and chewed) or smoked in a pipe. An elevated temperature, such as that provided with a butane torch, is usually preferred for burning the leaves.

4. *What is the timeline from ingestion to peak effect to a return to a pre-ingestion state?*
The timeline of Salvia's effects depends on the route of ingestion, since chewing and smoking timelines are different. Chewing the leaf brings its effects on more slowly, usually over a period of 10–15 minutes and lasting for 40–50 minutes. The bitter taste of the leaves usually prevents individuals from chewing for extended periods, i.e., long enough to obtain a psychedelic effect. If Salvia is smoked, the effects are experienced quickly, with peak effects reached within a minute and lasting for 1–5 minutes. Around the 10-minute mark, some effects usually persist, and normalcy returns after around twenty minutes.

5. *What are some of the effects of ingesting Salvia?*
The effects of Salvia include:

Improved mood
Calmness
Weird thoughts
Unreal thinking
Floating feeling
Sweating

        Warm feeling
        Increased self-confidence
6. *What ECG is the patient presenting with?*
    The patient is presenting in a sinus dysrhythmia.
7. *How do people usually feel after the drug has worn off?*
    Once the drug has worn off, people usually feel irritable. They may have extreme pain and a headache or feel as if they are being torn in half. They may also have little recollection of the entire incident.

Chapter 19
Hematology

Hematology is the study of blood and blood-formed organs. Blood disorders are common but rarely a primary medical emergency in EMS calls. Such disorders may include hemophilia, sickle cell anemia, hepatitis, or HIV. Patients with hematological disorders often complain of signs and symptoms that do not point to their primary cause. Through a thorough history-taking and assessment, the paramedic may be able to determine what impact such disorders may be having on a patient's presentation.

CASE 19.1

You are dispatched on a hot summer's day to 1234 Seaway, St. John's, Newfoundland, for a seven-year-old boy with a bleeding nose. On arrival you are met by the boy's mother, who tells you that her son Devon was playing outside and came into the house when his nose started to bleed. Devon told her that he did not bang himself; the nosebleed started on its own. She has been pinching his nose to stop the bleeding for the past 30 minutes, but it hasn't stopped. She reports that she even applied ice without success. She is very apologetic. Devon is beside his mom, who is still pinching his nose. He says hello and is very polite.

Initial Assessment Findings & Chief Complaint

LOA	Conscious and alert.
A	Patent with dried blood around mouth.
B	Regular and full volume.
C	Strong radial pulse present.
Wet Check	Ongoing epistaxis.
CC	Epistaxis.

History

S	Epistaxis ongoing for one hour.
A	None.
M	None.
P	Healthy.
L	Eating throughout the day.
E	The patient was playing outside when he had a sudden onset of a nosebleed. The patient's mother has been trying to stop the bleeding for over an hour without success.

Assessment

H/N	Unremarkable, with the exception of an ongoing nosebleed.
Chest	Unremarkable, with equal air entry bilaterally.
ABD	Soft/non-tender.
Back	Unremarkable.
Pelvis	Stable.
Ext	Deep bruises noted on the patient's upper and lower legs. Equal strength and mobility in all extremities. Capillary refill normal.

Vitals

BP	106/68
P	75, regular
RR	16
Pupils	PERL 3+ mm
GCS	4+5+6=15
BS	4.8 mmol/l
Pulse oximetry	100%
Skin	Warm, dry

Pain Assessment

O	n/a
P	n/a
Q	n/a
R	n/a
S	n/a
T	n/a

Cardiac Monitor

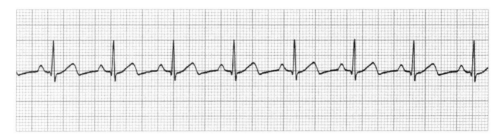

Figure 19.1

Initial Treatment Post Assessment

The patient should be assessed while pressure is held to his nose in an attempt to stop the bleeding. A complete set of vitals should be obtained, including an ECG interpretation. The pressure should be released in order to reassess the rate of bleeding. When released, blood may continue to trickle, and if so, the patient should blow his nose to clear it and pressure should once again be applied. He should be transported to the hospital in a sitting position.

En route, the patient's nosebleed does not stop. Devon's nose has now been bleeding for approximately one hour. He complains of nausea and is frustrated that he has to go to the hospital.

Treatment Continued

Ongoing pressure should be applied to Devon's nose, and he should expectorate the blood instead of swallowing it. Vitals should be monitored en route to the hospital. An intravenous should be established and infused at TKVO.

Differential Diagnosis

- Epistaxis.
- Underlying clotting disorder.

Test Your Knowledge

1. Why has the epistaxis not been successfully stopped?
2. What is hemophilia?
3. Why does a patient with hemophilia take longer to stop bleeding?
4. What are common bleeding manifestations in patients with hemophilia?
5. What are typical signs and symptoms of hemophilia?
6. While adults often know they are hemophiliacs, children may not have been diagnosed. When should hemophilia be suspected in children?
7. What ECG is the patient presenting with?

CASE 19.2

You are dispatched to 175 Third Avenue, Fort MacLeod, Alberta, for a 27-year-old male complaining of severe abdominal pain. It is a cool April morning and it finally stops raining as you pull up to the residence. You knock on the door and are greeted by a young woman who tells you that her husband Ajala is lying on the bed upstairs. She says he is in too much pain to move. She reports that this is the second episode since January and her husband is fed up. This time the pain is in his lower abdomen and groin. As you walk into the bedroom, you see the patient lying with his knees to his chest on the bed.

Initial Assessment Findings & Chief Complaint

LOA	Conscious and alert.
A	Patent.
B	Regular and full volume.
C	Strong radial pulse.
Wet Check	Unremarkable.
CC	Abdominal and groin pain.

History

S	Complaining of pain increasing in severity over the past several hours.
A	None.
M	Tylenol, Pulmicort, salbutamol.
P	sickle cell disease, asthma.
L	Egg and muffin at breakfast.
E	The patient is complaining of ongoing pain increasing in severity since this morning. The pain is located in his lower abdomen, groin, and penis/scrotum.

Assessment

H/N	Unremarkable.
Chest	Unremarkable with expiratory wheezing present in the apexes bilaterally.
ABD	Severe pain increasing on palpation to the RLQ, radiating into the groin. Pain present in scrotum and penis, with priapism.
Back	Unremarkable.
Pelvis	Stable.
Ext	Equal strength and mobility in all extremities.

Vitals

BP	130/88
P	150, regular
RR	20
Pupils	PERL 3+ mm
GCS	4+5+6=15
BS	n/a
Pulse oximetry	100%
Skin	Warm, diaphoretic

Pain Assessment

O	Gradual
P	While at rest, throughout the day
Q	Sharp
R	To groin
S	10/10
T	5 hours

Cardiac Monitor

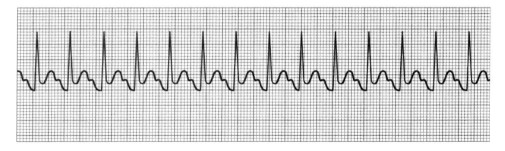

Figure 19.2

Initial Treatment Post Assessment

The patient should be assessed and a complete set of vitals obtained, including ECG interpretation. Oxygen should be administered via a high concentration mask, and salbutamol administered via MDI according to local protocols. An intravenous should be initiated and infused at TKVO. An ACP should not administer analgesics until a diagnosis has been confirmed.

En route to the hospital, the patient's breathing is improving and he is no longer wheezing in the apexes. He still complains of severe pain in the groin as well as priapism.

Treatment Continued

Ongoing assessment of the patient should continue, as should supportive care. Oxygen should continue to be administered and the patient should be placed in a position of comfort.

Differential Diagnosis

- Vasoocclusive pain crisis associated with SCD.
- Asthma.

Test Your Knowledge

1. What is sickle cell disease?
2. What are common signs and symptoms of sickle cell disease?
3. What is a vasoocclusive pain crisis?
4. What are typical emergencies in sickle cell disease?
5. What ECG is the patient presenting in?

Answers

Case 19.1

1. *Why has the epistaxis not been successfully stopped?*

   Success in stopping Devon's epistaxis has not been achieved because of a possible bleeding disorder which has not yet been diagnosed.

2. *What is hemophilia?*

   Hemophilia is a bleeding disorder of coagulation caused primarily by a deficiency or defect in one of the two plasma proteins. The most common factor abnormalities are factor VIII or factor IX.

3. *Why does a patient with hemophilia take longer to stop bleeding?*

   The hemophiliac patient takes longer to stop bleeding because of a lack of plasma proteins. Normal hemostatic mechanisms of platelet aggregation and vasoconstriction still occur, but plugging will not be stable.

4. *What are common bleeding manifestations in patients with hemophilia?*

   Common bleeding manifestations in patients with hemophilia include:

Hemarthroses	May lead to joint destruction
Hematomas	Soft tissue bleeding
Mucocutaneous bleeding	Dental extraction bleeding
CNS	Intracranial bleeding
Hematuria	Bleeding source not found
Pseudotumours	Bone cysts

5. *What are typical signs and symptoms of hemophilia?*

   Typical signs and symptoms of hemophilia may include:
   - Easy bruising
   - Hemarthrosis
   - Deep muscle bleeding
   - Pain (pulled muscle feeling)
   - Unusual bleeding

6. *While adults often know they are hemophiliacs, children may not have been diagnosed. When should hemophilia be suspected in children?*

   Hemophilia should be suspected in any child that presents with spontaneous bleeding, excessive bruising, or bleeding into the joints, muscles, or central nervous system that may be out of proportion to the patient's history or mechanism of injury.

7. *What ECG is the patient presenting with?*

   The patient is presenting in a normal sinus rhythm.

Case 19.2

1. *What is sickle cell disease?*

   Sickle cell disease is a disorder that affects red blood cells. Sickle cell anemia patients have hemoglobin that differs from normal hemoglobin. Normal red blood cells can move and bend freely, while sickle hemoglobin sticks together to form rigid rods inside red blood cells. This makes red blood cells more fragile and at risk of rupturing. With their changed shape, sickle red blood cells may not squeeze through small blood vessels and may occlude them. Sickle cell disease is inherited and primarily affects people of African, Asian, or Caribbean descent.

2. *What are common signs and symptoms of sickle cell disease (SCD)?*

   Common signs and symptoms of sickle cell disease may include:

   Fatigue
   Anemia
   Dactylitis
   Bacterial infections
   Leg ulcers
   Eye damage
   Pain crises

3. *What is a vasoocclusive pain crisis?*

   A vasoocclusive pain crisis is an acutely painful sickle crisis, and is a common problem for patients with SCD. Most SCD patients have an average of four severe attacks per year. Usually they will present as diffuse bone, muscle, or joint pain caused by small blood vessel occlusion.

4. *What are typical emergencies in sickle cell disease?*

   Typical emergencies in SCD include:

   Vasoocclusive crises
   Musculoskeletal pain
   Dactylitis
   Priapism
   Chest pain

   Hematologic crises
   Splenic sequestration
   Aplastic crises
   Infections
   Pneumonia
   Meningitis
   Sepsis
   UTI

5. *What ECG is the patient presenting in?*

   The patient is presenting in a sinus tachycardia.

Chapter 20
Environmental Emergencies

Canadians are exposed to vast extremes of weather, have access to fresh and salt water, and live and work in terrain ranging from arctic to desert-like conditions. Environmental emergencies are conditions caused or exacerbated by exposure to such environments. These may include cold or heat exposure, elevation exposure, diving, or drowning. Environmental emergencies can affect anyone, but pose particular risks for the elderly and the very young, and for those with poor general health, fatigue, and predisposing medical conditions. The paramedic's primary goal is to remove patients from negative environments. Minimizing exposure to extreme conditions may also be a concern for an EMS. A thorough incident history, including a timeline and assessment, will improve a patient's outcome.

CASE 20.1

You are dispatched to Highway 144, north of the Gogama Watershed, Ontario, for a possible drowning. It is early spring and the weather is just beginning to improve after the long winter, with the temperature around 18°C. However, your response time will be considerable: it is raining and lightning has made air transport impossible. Your estimated time of arrival is 20 minutes. When you arrive at the scene, you are greeted by several teenagers who tell you that Matt, a 19-year-old friend, was cliff-jumping with the rest of the group and didn't come up after diving into the water. When Matt didn't surface immediately, his friends brought him to shore. They tell you he was out cold and not breathing. One of the friends, who knows CPR, initiated rescue breathing. After about a minute, Matt started to breathe and has been breathing ever since, though in a laboured fashion.

Initial Assessment Findings & Chief Complaint

LOA	Unresponsive.
A	Patent.
B	Shallow with audible congestion.
C	Weak radial pulse.
Wet Check	Skin wet, cold in the extremities.
CC	Unconscious, respiratory distress.

History

S	Patient unresponsive with respiratory depression.
A	CNO.
M	Seizure medications, according to friends.
P	Seizure disorder.
L	Breakfast.
E	The teenager and his friends shared a 26-oz bottle of vodka and began cliff-jumping. The water was extremely cold, so they were just jumping in and out. The patient, Matt, dove in but didn't come up, and his friends pulled him from the water. His head was bleeding when they removed him and he was not breathing. However, a friend began AR and the patient started to breathe. Matt's friends called 911 as soon as they pulled him from the water, and he is now covered with blankets.

Assessment

H/N	Approximately 3-cm laceration superior to left eye; bleeding has stopped.
Chest	Symmetrical, air entry decreased with crackles throughout.
ABD	Soft, slightly distended.
Back	Unremarkable.
Pelvis	Stable.
Ext	Unremarkable, pale and cool to touch.

Vitals

BP	86/46
P	38, regular
RR	8
Pupils	PERL 4 mm, slow to react
GCS	1+1+1=3
BS	5.4 mmol/l
Pulse oximetry	90%
Skin	Cool extremities, pale, damp

Pain Assessment

O	n/a
P	n/a
Q	n/a
R	n/a
S	n/a
T	n/a

Cardiac Monitor

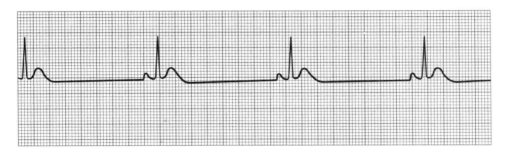

Figure 20.1

Initial Treatment Post Assessment

Cervical spine control should be maintained during assessment because of the mechanism of injury. Adequate suctioning of the patient's airway should be performed, and an airway adjunct such as an OPA, combitube, or LMA should be inserted. An ACP should intubate the patient because of his decreased GCS. Care should also be taken to perform in-line stabilization because of the potential for spinal or head injury. The patient should then be adequately oxygenated to improve perfusion. Cardiac monitoring should be continued throughout the call and transport to hospital. A blood glucometry and complete set of vitals should also be obtained. As well, a cervical collar should be applied and the patient placed on a spinal board for spinal immobilization. If possible, the head of the stretcher should be elevated slightly to facilitate drainage en route to the hospital. Once in the vehicle, the patient's wet clothing should be removed and hot packs placed on his groin, axillary regions, and behind his head. A dressing should be applied to the head laceration.

Differential Diagnosis

- Near drowning.
- Head/spinal injury.

Test Your Knowledge

1. What is important to obtain from the bystanders?
2. What ECG rhythm is the patient presenting with?

3. There are two types of drowning. What are they and how do they differ?
4. What are possible complications of drowning?
5. What is the typical sequence of events in a drowning or near-drowning?
6. What is frequently a contributing factor to drowning?
7. How does saltwater drowning differ from freshwater drowning?

CASE 20.2

At close to 20:00hrs on an evening in mid-July, you are dispatched to Kejimkujik Park, Nova Scotia, for a patient who is not feeling well. Temperatures have been hovering around 35°C for the past several days. You can't wait to finish the night; it is your last shift before heading to Ontario for a week's holiday. As you approach the scene, you are met by two or three bystanders who tell you they have been hiking for the past two days and were almost back at the rally point when one of them, Brandon, collapsed to the ground and began shaking. You observe that they each have large backpacks with sleeping gear and camping equipment.

Initial Assessment Findings & Chief Complaint

LOA	Decreased level of awareness.
A	Patent.
B	Shallow, regular.
C	Barely palpable radial pulse.
Wet Check	Incontinent of urine.
CC	Collapse, possible seizure.

History

S	Patient is semi-conscious and very hot to the touch, with dry mucous membranes.
A	penicillin, environmental.
M	Claritin.
P	No health issues.
L	Around lunch time, protein bar (the last of the food).
E	The group was just finishing a 30-km hike that had begun that morning. For the past hour, Brandon had been complaining of nausea, as had everyone else: they had not eaten much throughout the day. About half an hour earlier, according to his companions, Brandon started making weird comments and talking nonsense. At times he even walked off the trail and had to be redirected. As the group approached the car, Brandon collapsed. The group thought he was just tired until he started twitching and could not be roused. The friends called 911, and it has taken approximately 15 minutes for the medics to arrive.

Assessment

H/N	No JVD, trachea midline, dry mucous membranes, chapped lips.
Chest	Unremarkable, hot to touch under shirt. Patient's shirt is dry.
ABD	Soft/non-tender.
Back	Unremarkable, hot to touch.
Pelvis	Stable.
Ext	Unremarkable, minor abrasions on legs and hands from the trip.

Vitals

BP	78/58
P	30, regular
RR	12
Pupils	PERL 4 mm, slow
GCS	2+3+4=9
BS	4.1 mmol/l
Pulse oximetry	93%
Skin	Hot, dry to touch

Pain Assessment

O	n/a
P	n/a
Q	n/a
R	n/a
S	n/a
T	n/a

Cardiac Monitor

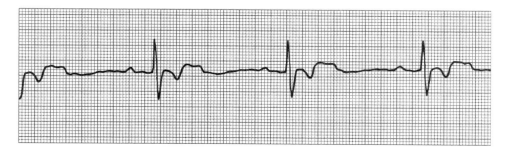

Figure 20.2

Initial Treatment Post Assessment

The patient's airway should be assessed post-seizure, and an NPA inserted with oxygen administered via a high concentration mask. After an assessment, vitals and a blood glucometry should be obtained. The patient's clothing should be removed and he should be transported to the ambulance. Cooling should then be initiated with cold packs to the patient's axillary regions, groin, neck, and head in an attempt to decrease his body temperature. An intravenous should be started and a fluid bolus initiated at 20 ml/kg to maintain a blood pressure of 100 systolic. Nothing should be given to the patient by mouth. Continuous ECG and vital signs monitoring should be performed en route to the hospital.

En route, the patient's body begins to cool and he appears more awake with a GCS of 4+4+5=13. His vitals are: BP 110/60, radial pulse of 75 and regular, respirations full volume at 16, PERL 3+ mm, and SPO2 99%. His ECG is as follows.

Cardiac Monitor

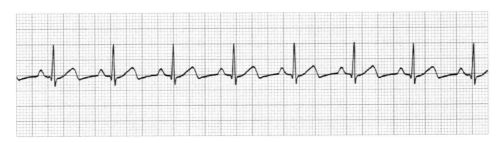

Figure 20.3

Treatment Continued

The fluid bolus should be discontinued and the IV infused at TKVO. Cooling should be maintained throughout transport if travel time is less than 30 minutes to ensure the patient's body temperature does not elevate. If his body temperature feels normal to the touch or shivering begins, cooling should be discontinued.

Differential Diagnosis

- Heatstroke.

Test Your Knowledge

1. Why and when does heatstroke occur?
2. What are the typical signs and symptoms of heatstroke?
3. Why does sweating stop in heatstroke?
4. What is the difference between classic and exertional heatstroke?
5. What other condition goes hand in hand with heatstroke?
7. What ECG rhythm is the patient presenting with?
8. What is heat exhaustion?

CASE 20.3

Around 09:30hrs, you are dispatched to a groomed snow-machine trail at the north end of Sexsmith, Alberta, for a possible unconscious patient. Upon arrival, you are greeted by a group on snow machines. One of the members of the group approaches and informs you that several friends spent the previous night at a camp approximately two kilometres up the trail, where they had a little party celebrating the coming of spring. He tells you that 18-year-old Joe, who had plenty to drink, wandered off around 02:00hrs. After looking for him in the dark, they found him lying on the trail at about 06:00hrs this morning. Joe's friend tells you that the patient is cold and that they covered him up on the trail where they found him. Knowing how cold it was on your way to work this morning, you estimate it must have been at least -15°C overnight. You board a snow machine with a sled attached and venture down the trail. As you approach, you see the patient lying on the ground in a fetal position covered with blankets, with several others standing around him.

Initial Assessment Findings & Chief Complaint

LOA	Patient appears disoriented and gazes through you as you introduce yourself.
A	Airway appears patent.
B	Shallow at approximately 10.
C	Weak radial pulse, slow and hard to count.
Wet Check	Unremarkable.
CC	Exposure.

History

S	Patient appears disoriented and rigid with uncoordinated movements and minimal shivering as you remove the blankets. He is wearing a hoodie, jeans, and running shoes.
A	CNO.
M	CNO.
P	MedicAlert necklace for epilepsy.
L	According to friends, they ate hot dogs around the fire around 22:00hrs.
E	Joe was drinking with his friends when an argument developed and he walked away from the party down the skidoo trail. The friends assumed he had gone back to the camp but around 03:30hrs they could not find him and began a search. When they found him, they called 911. The friends tell you that Joe drank approximately 26 ounces of vodka and smoked some marijuana last night.

Assessment

H/N	White chalky appearance.
Chest	Unremarkable, cold to touch with equal air entry bilaterally.
ABD	Soft/non-tender.
Back	Unremarkable, cold to touch.
Pelvis	Stable.
Ext	Uncoordinated movement in the upper extremities, cold to touch with obvious frostbite on all fingers of the left hand and on ring and middle fingers of the right hand.

Vitals

BP	76/58
P	38 weak (femoral)
RR	10 shallow
Pupils	PERL 5 mm, slow
GCS	3+3+4=10
BS	4.1 mmol/l
Pulse oximetry	91%
Skin	Pale, white, cold to touch

Pain Assessment

O	n/a
P	n/a
Q	n/a
R	n/a
S	n/a
T	n/a

Cardiac Monitor

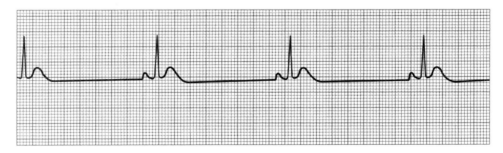

Figure 20.4

Initial Treatment Post Assessment

The patient's ABCs should be assessed and a quick primary survey completed on the trail including mechanisms of injury, ruling out trauma and c-spine protection. A baseline set of vitals and blood glucometry should be completed on scene. The patient should then be placed carefully on a stretcher and moved to the rescue sled. He should be covered with several blankets. Foil blankets may also be used during transport to the warm awaiting vehicle. Once inside, oxygen should be administered via a high concentration mask and a cardiac monitor applied. An attempt to raise the temperature of the oxygen by wrapping the tubing in hot packs may be beneficial for the patient. Clothing should be removed to warm the patient and to allow a more detailed assessment. An intravenous should be initiated and a 20 ml/kg bolus started to maintain a blood pressure of 100/P. The IV tubing could be wrapped around a hot pack to warm the administered fluid. All jewelry and rings should be removed if possible, and the patient should be placed in a position of comfort.

En route to the hospital, Joe has greater coordination of his upper extremities and is becoming more aware of his surroundings. He is still confused as to what happened the previous night but is able to communicate with you. His vitals are BP 110/78, P 75, RR 18, SPO2 98%, GCS 4+4+6=14, and his skin is warmer and less white. The patient is now shivering and tells you he is getting warmer.

Cardiac Monitor

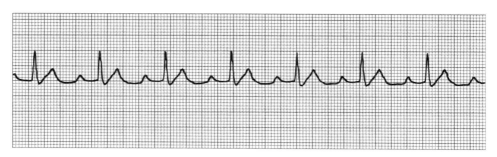

Figure 20.5

Treatment Continued

En route, the IV rate can be decreased to TKVO. Morphine sulphate or fentanyl can be administered to ease the pain of hypothermia in the patient's hands. The patient should be monitored during transport, with ongoing reassessment of his core temperature. Hot packs should now be applied to the groin, axillary regions, and behind the neck.

Differential Diagnosis

- Hypothermia.

Test Your Knowledge

1. Hypothermia is considered to occur at what body temperature?
2. What are the typical signs and symptoms of mild hypothermia?
3. What are the typical signs and symptoms of severe hypothermia?
4. At what temperature does shivering cease?
5. Without a thermometer, what patient action can help the paramedic differentiate between severe and mild hypothermia?
6. What ECG is the patient presenting in?
7. What is a typical ECG tracing found in patients suffering from hypothermia?
8. What is the treatment for Joe's frostbitten hands and fingers?

CASE 20.4

You are dispatched to Departure Bay, British Columbia, for a possible unconscious patient. You recognize the place name as a popular scuba diving location. As you arrive, you see a few young guys sitting on the shoreline. Montana approaches and tells you that he and his friend Kim, who is 16 years old, borrowed his dad's scuba gear for the afternoon. Neither had dived before, but Kim had seen his dad do it and figured it couldn't be too hard. The diving went fine, and they called it quits after approximately 45 minutes. They chilled on the shore for another hour until Kim started complaining of pain.

Initial Assessment Findings & Chief Complaint

LOA	Conscious and alert.
A	Patent.
B	Regular and full volume.
C	Strong radial pulses.
Wet Check	Unremarkable.
CC	Shoulder pain.

History

S	The patient is complaining of an onset of a deep pain in the left shoulder.
A	Pine nuts.
M	Tetracycline.
P	Healthy.
L	Breakfast.
E	The friends were diving and came out of the water after approximately one hour. Some time later, the patient complained of severe shoulder pain. He denies any trauma to the shoulder or extremities. When asked, the patient says he was diving at approximately 13–14 m and raced to the surface quickly to get out of the water.

Assessment

H/N	No JVD, trachea midline.
Chest	Unremarkable, with equal air entry bilaterally.
ABD	Soft/non-tender.
Back	Unremarkable.
Pelvis	Stable.
Ext	Equal strength and mobility, with good peripheral circulation and capillary refill. Pain in left shoulder not agitated or eased by movement.

Vitals

BP	110/70
P	68, irregular
RR	18
Pupils	PERL 3+ mm
GCS	4+5+6=15
BS	n/a
Pulse oximetry	100%
Skin	Warm, dry

Pain Assessment

O	Sudden
P	Diving for 45 minutes
Q	Sharp, deep
R	None
S	8/10
T	1 hour

Cardiac Monitor

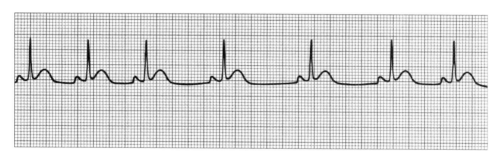

Figure 20.6

Initial Treatment Post Assessment

The patient should be assessed and vitals obtained, including pulse oximetry and an ECG. Oxygen should be administered via a high concentration mask. Details of the dive, including specifics of the length, time, and depth of descent of the dive should be obtained. The patient should be transported in a position of comfort to the hospital. There is no treatment specific to ACPs for this patient.

En route, the patient continues to complain of left shoulder pain.

Differential Diagnosis

- Decompression illness (the bends).

Test Your Knowledge

1. What are important questions to be asked in regards to the dive?
2. Is decompression illness an injury related to the surface, descent, bottom, or ascent of a dive?
3. In a case of the bends, where is pain usually located?

4. What is the classification of patient's medication?
5. What causes decompression sickness or the bends?
6. What is the difference between type I and type II DCS?
7. Why does treatment of the bends include positioning the patient in a left lateral recumbent position?

Answers
Case 20.1

1. *What is important to obtain from the bystanders?*

   On arrival, it is important to find out the mechanism of injury of the incident. In this particular case, it is imperative to ask:

   Did Matt jump or dive headfirst or feet-first into the water?
   How deep is the water?
   How long was he under the water before he was brought to the surface?
   How long before he started to breathe?
   Did he vomit before he started to breathe?
   How much alcohol has Matt ingested?

2. *What ECG rhythm is the patient presenting with?*

   The patient is presenting with a sinus bradycardia.

3. *There are two types of drowning. What are they and how do they differ?*

   The two types of drowning are wet and dry drowning. In wet drowning, a significant amount of water enters the lungs, leading to hemodilution and hypoxemia. In dry drowning, during the panic phase the patient inhales a mouthful of water, which stimulates laryngospasm. Laryngospasm prevents further aspiration of water but also leads to hypoxia and unconsciousness. It accounts for approximately 10 percent of drownings and an even greater percentage of near-drownings.

4. *What are possible complications of drowning?*

   Some of the complications of drowning include hypothermia, aspiration, pulmonary edema, and possible trauma associated with the incident.

5. *What is the typical sequence of events in a drowning or near-drowning?*

   The typical sequence of events in a drowning includes:

   A patient is submerged in water.
   If conscious, the patient undergoes complete apnea for a period of up to three minutes.
   Blood is shunted to the core because of the mammalian dive reflex.
   PCO2 increases and PO2 decreases, resulting in hypoxia and stimulation from the CNS.

6. *What is frequently a contributing factor of drowning?*

   Alcohol use is frequently a contributing factor in drowning and near-drowning cases, both by the victim and by adults supervising inexperienced swimmers or children.

7. *How does saltwater drowning differ from freshwater drowning?*

   There are unique differences between freshwater and saltwater drowning. In freshwater drowning, which could happen in most parts of Canada, hypotonic water is diffused across the alveoli into vascular spaces. This results in hemodilution as well as inflammatory responses and destruction of surfactant. Atelectasis is a result of hemodilution and shunts unoxygenated blood back into circulation. Hypoxemia from pulmonary edema is the end result. In saltwater drowning, hypertonic sea water, draws water from the bloodstream into the alveoli, producing more volume in the lungs. This type of drowning also results in hypoxemia from pulmonary edema and the shunting of unoxygenated blood into circulation.

Case 20.2

1. *Why and when does heatstroke occur?*

   Heatstroke normally occurs when the body temperature is at least 40.6°C, and usually when sweating ceases. It occurs because the body's thermoregulatory system fails, causing hyperthermia. Heatstroke may progress to cellular death and brain and kidney damage.

2. *What are the typical signs and symptoms of heatstroke?*

   The typical signs of heatstroke include:
   - Absence of sweating
   - Hot, dry skin (hot core)
   - Rapid pulses leading to slow pulses
   - Hypotension
   - Altered level of consciousness or unconsciousness
   - Syncope or seizures
   - Deep respirations

3. *Why does sweating stop in heatstroke?*

   Sensory overload causes the sweat glands to temporarily dysfunction. The patient's skin becomes hot even to the core.

4. *What is the difference between classic and exertional heatstroke?*

   Classic heatstroke is the result of illnesses that cause body temperature to increase because of poor thermoregulatory function. Exertional heatstroke tends to happen to those in good health who are exposed to excessive temperatures. In both cases, the skin will be hot to touch, although exertional heatstroke patients may have diaphoresis from previous heat exposure.

5. *What other condition goes hand in hand with heatstroke?*

   Dehydration is very common with heatstroke.

7. *What ECG rhythm is the patient presenting with?*

   The patient is presenting in a second-degree AV block, type 2, progressing to a normal sinus rhythm.

8. *What is heat exhaustion?*

   Heat exhaustion is a mild heat illness. It is very common and usually caused by physical exertion in a hot environment. The patient will lose water and sodium through sweating, and will then present as if they have lost circulating volume, i.e., with symptoms such as tachycardia, skin that is cool and clammy, and tachypnea.

Case 20.3

1. *Hypothermia is considered to occur at what body temperature?*

   Hypothermia can be divided into two categories: Mild, with body temperatures > 32°C; and severe, with body temperatures < 32°C.

2. *What are the typical signs and symptoms of mild hypothermia?*

   Typical signs of mild hypothermia include:
   - Shivering
   - Confusion
   - Lack of coordination

Pale, dry, cold skin
Rise in BP and heart rate

3. *What are the typical signs and symptoms of severe hypothermia?*

    Typical signs of severe hypothermia include:

    Loss of shivering
    Decrease in pulse and respirations
    Loss of voluntary muscle movement
    Uncoordinated muscle movement
    Dysrhythmias
    Asystole
    Hypotension
    VSA

4. *At what temperature does shivering cease?*

    Shivering ceases at approximately 32°C.

5. *Without a thermometer, what patient action can help the paramedic differentiate between severe and mild hypothermia?*

    If shivering is minimal or absent and the patient's level of consciousness is decreased, you may assume that the body's core temperature is less than 32°C.

6. *What ECG is the patient presenting in?*

    The patient is presenting in a sinus bradycardia progressing to a first-degree AV block.

7. *What is a typical ECG tracing found in patients suffering from hypothermia?*

    A J-wave or Osborne wave may be seen in patients suffering from hypothermia. This type of wave is a deflection found at the junction of the QRS and ST segments.

8. *What is the treatment for Joe's frostbitten hands and fingers?*

    The frostbitten areas should not be thawed if there is a possibility of them refreezing. Allow the areas to passively thaw by covering them with dry, sterile dressings. The affected areas should be elevated and blisters should not be broken.

Case 20.4

1. *What are important questions to be asked in regards to the dive?*

    As a paramedic, there are several questions that you should ask regarding the dive.

    When did the symptoms occur?
    What were the parameters of the dive, including, depth, length, and number of dives?
    What was the rate of ascent, and was it controlled or panic-forced?
    Was the patient an experienced or an inexperienced diver?
    Have there been previous episodes of decompression illness?
    Did the incident involve the ingestion of alcohol or drugs?

2. *Is decompression illness an injury related to the surface, descent, bottom, or ascent of a dive?*

    Decompression illness is related to the ascent of a dive.

3. *In a case of the bends, where is pain usually located?*

    In a case of decompression illness or the bends, the patient usually complains of a deep pain in the knees or shoulders. Usually a single joint is involved.

4. *What is the classification of the patient's medication?*

    tetracycline (Tetracyn) — Antibiotic

5. **What causes decompression sickness or the bends?**

   Decompression sickness (DCS) or the bends is caused by a rapid ascent from 12 m or more. It is related to the obstructive and inflammatory effects of inert gas bubbles in tissues. DCS occurs when divers are subjected to a rapid reduction in air pressure during an ascent, after being exposed to compressed air.

6. **What is the difference between type I and type II DCS?**

   Type I DCS is associated with pain in the joints that is unrelieved but not worsened by movement. Type II DCS includes neurological involvement and affects the spinal cord in compressed air divers. Type II symptoms include girdle-like pain and a paresthesia or paralysis of the feet.

7. **Why does treatment of the bends include positioning the patient in a left lateral recumbent position?**

   This position was originally thought to trap or isolate air in the ventricle if physical signs and symptoms suggest an arterial gas embolism (AGE). By the time a patient is transported by ambulance, the air has usually been distributed throughout the body. Oxygen administration and placing the patient in a position of comfort is the pre-hospital treatment for the bends.

8. **What ECG is the patient presenting in?**

   The patient is presenting in a sinus dysrhythmia.

Chapter 21
Infectious Disease

Infectious diseases are illnesses caused by biological organisms such as bacteria and viruses. While most infectious diseases are not life-threatening, some—such as HIV, hepatitis B, and bacterial meningitis—can be fatal. Paramedics must maintain a strong working knowledge of infectious diseases and be current with treatment and prevention strategies. As paramedics are in close contact with patients in confined areas, they must take some precautions. This is of paramount importance in cases involving the possible exchange of body fluids such as blood.

CASE 21.1

You are dispatched mid-morning to 281 Thurlow Street, Vancouver, for an unwell female. On arrival you are greeted by Hatsuyo, aged 36. She tells you she has not been feeling well for the past several weeks and feels worse today. She looks sick, as if she has not been eating well, and is short of breath. Hatsuyo says she works at Canada Customs and has been off work for a week, but today was the breaking point. She has not seen her doctor since she thought she would get better, but she hasn't improved. She complains of fever, general malaise, and coughing that started weeks ago. She is now coughing so badly that she complains of pain in her chest wall. Her sputum is blood-tinged.

Initial Assessment Findings & Chief Complaint

LOA	Conscious and alert.
A	Patent.
B	Shallow with coughing bouts.
C	Strong, radial.
Wet Check	Unremarkable.
CC	Unwell for three weeks with a cough.

History

S	Complains of shortness of breath with productive cough and fever.
A	monk fish.
M	Zestoretic, Buckley's.
P	Mild hypertension.
L	Breakfast: rice pudding and tea.
E	The patient has been unwell for several weeks and complains of weight loss, fever, a productive cough with hemoptysis, shortness of breath, and general malaise. She has tried several over-the-counter medications without success. She has been home from work for a week and was to return today, but her symptoms have worsened.

Assessment

H/N	No JVD, trachea midline.
Chest	Unremarkable, shallow respirations with equal air entry.
ABD	Soft/non-tender.
Back	Unremarkable.
Pelvis	Stable.
Ext	Weak bilaterally upper and lower, with equal distal pulses present.

Vitals

BP	98/78
P	70, irregular
RR	22 shallow
Pupils	PERL 3+ mm
GCS	4+5+6=15
BS	4.2.mmol/l
Pulse oximetry	96%
Skin	Warm, dry

Pain Assessment

O	Gradual
P	Coughing
Q	Sore
R	None
S	Unable to assign any specific number
T	Ongoing

Cardiac Monitor

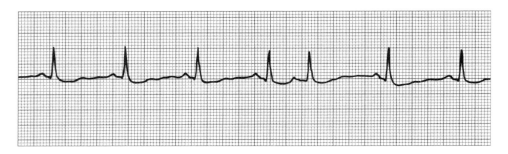

Figure 21.1

Initial Treatment Post Assessment

An initial assessment should be completed and a complete set of vitals obtained, including SPO2 and blood glucometry. The patient should be administered oxygen via a high concentration mask. Based on the febrile state of the patient and her productive cough, the paramedic should be wearing an N95 mask as well as all other PPE deemed appropriate. The patient's breathing should be assessed and administration of a bronchodilator, e.g., salbutamol, may be of assistance. The patient should be transported in a position of comfort on a stretcher. There are no significant treatment differences between a PCP and an ACP.

En route to the hospital, the patient feels less winded but still has a productive cough and complains of weakness.

Differential Diagnosis

- Respiratory infection with the possibility of tuberculosis (TB).

Test Your Knowledge

1. What may increase Hatsuyo's susceptibility to contracting communicable diseases?
2. What are the common signs and symptoms of TB?

3. Among what patients may TB be more prevalent?
4. When transporting the patient to the hospital, what else can be done to limit the paramedic's exposure?
5. What are the classifications of the patient's medications?
6. What ECG is the patient presenting with?
7. What do most EMS agencies require of paramedics on an annual basis?

CASE 21.2

You are dispatched at 15:45hrs to 120 King Street, Grand Falls, New Brunswick, for a possible seizure. On arrival, you are summoned to a bedroom where you find a mother and daughter. The mother, Sara, tells you that her five-year-old daughter, Brianna, has had a seizure. Sara says it seemed to last for about 30 seconds and stopped right after she got off the phone with the emergency dispatcher. Sara is quite concerned as her daughter has had an ear infection and now a seizure. She says Brianna was healthy up to this point except for the last week. Today she seemed to mope around the house and complained of a headache. The daughter opens her eyes and recognizes your presence.

Initial Assessment Findings & Chief Complaint

LOA	Conscious.
A	Patent.
B	Full volume at 20.
C	Strong radial pulses.
Wet Check	Unremarkable.
CC	Seizure.

History

S	Lethargic, not herself.
A	None.
M	Amoxil, Tempra.
P	None. Family history of diabetes.
L	Lunch (soup).
E	Mother states that the child has been sick for a week with an earache. Brianna complained earlier today of a headache but the mother thought it was because of the ear infection. Brianna went to bed and shortly afterward had a 30-second-long seizure.

Assessment

H/N	Unremarkable, but pain on palpation of occiput.
Chest	Unremarkable, equal air entry bilaterally with no adventitious sounds.
ABD	Soft/non-tender.
Back	Unremarkable.
Pelvis	Stable.
Ext	Equal strength and mobility in upper and lower extremities.

Vitals   Pain Assessment

BP	106/68	O	Gradual
P	70, regular	P	At rest
RR	20	Q	Constant ache
Pupils	PERL 3+ mm	R	None
GCS	4+5+6=15	S	Hurts a lot
BS	5.8 mmol/l	T	All day
Pulse oximetry	100%		
Skin	Warm, dry		

Cardiac Monitor

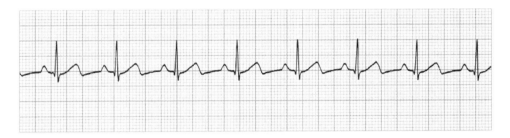

Figure 21.2

Initial Treatment Post Assessment

The patient should be assessed and oxygen administered via a high concentration mask. A complete set of vitals should be obtained, including SPO2 and blood glucometry. The patient should be placed on a stretcher in a position of comfort. An intravenous should be secured and maintained at TKVO. The mother should escort the child to the hospital in the ambulance.

En route, the patient is crying and complains of a more severe headache.

Treatment Continued

The cabin lights should be dimmed and the child reassessed en route. A complete set of vitals should be obtained. The child should be comforted and reassured.

Differential Diagnosis

- Meningitis.

Test Your Knowledge

1. What is meningitis?
2. What is the typical cause of meningitis?
3. What are the typical signs and symptoms of meningitis?
4. What two signs may be positive with meningitis?
5. What ECG is the patient presenting with?
6. How may infants present with meningitis?
7. What is the classification of the patient's medication?

Answers

Case 21.1

1. *What may increase Hatsuyo's susceptibility to contracting communicable diseases?*

    Hatsuyo's exposure to infectious and communicable diseases is increased because of her work environment. She is exposed on a daily basis to many people who have travelled from abroad and are re-entering Canada. Many travellers and tourists have underlying conditions they are unaware of or may have higher exposure rates to diseases. Communicable diseases can be spread not only by touch but also through airborne particles. Customs agents routinely wear gloves to help minimize the risk of contagion.

2. *What are the common signs and symptoms of TB?*

    The typical signs and symptoms of TB include:

    Non-specific symptoms
    Chills
    Fever
    Fatigue
    Weight loss
    Productive or non-productive cough
    Night sweats
    Shortness of breath
    Pleuritic chest pain

3. *Among what patients may TB be more prevalent?*

    TB may be more prevalent among the following kinds of patients:

    Elderly and nursing home patients
    Residents or staff of prisons or facilities for the homeless
    Alcoholics and illicit drug users
    Patients with HIV
    Immigrants from high exposure countries, or those exposed to them
    Patients from Northern Canada, where health care and immunizations are less readily available

4. *When transporting the patient to the hospital, what else can be done to limit the paramedic's exposure?*

    Universal precautions for the use of personal protective equipment should be initiated at all times during the call. If the patient is not in a respiratory-compromised state and will tolerate it, a mask can also be placed on the patient. Oxygen via nasal cannula can still be administered if the patient is wearing a mask.

5. *What are the classifications of the patient's medications?*

   Zestoretic (hydrochlorothiazide, lisinopril)   – ACEI, diuretic
   Buckley's (camphor or menthol)   – Non-alcohol, non-sugar cough syrup

6. *What ECG is the patient presenting with?*

   The patient is presenting in a normal sinus rhythm with premature atrial contractions.

7. *What do most EMS agencies require of paramedics on an annual basis?*

   Most EMS agencies require that paramedics obtain a TB test at least annually. This requirement is usually based on the prevalence of TB in a community.

Case 21.2

1. *What is meningitis?*

   Meningitis is an inflammation of the membranes protecting the brain, spinal cord, and cerebral spinal fluid, and can be caused by a bacterial or viral infection.

2. *What is the typical cause of meningitis?*

   The typical cause of meningitis, which is the most common risk to paramedics, is Neisseria meningitis.

3. *What are the typical signs and symptoms of meningitis?*

   The following signs and symptoms are typical of meningitis:

   Headache
   Nuchal rigidity with flexion
   Lethargy
   Malaise
   Altered mental status
   Fever
   Chills
   Vomiting
   Seizures

4. *What two signs may be positive with meningitis?*

   To test for Kernig's sign, the patient should sit or lie while flexing his or her hips. With the hips flexed, the patient should attempt to straighten the knee. The inability to straighten the knee is a positive Kernig's sign. Brudzinski's sign occurs when flexion of the neck also causes flexion of the hips and knees.

5. *What ECG is the patient presenting with?*

   The patient is presenting with a normal sinus rhythm.

6. *How may infants present with meningitis?*

   Infants with meningitis may present with:

   Slow or inactive behaviour
   Irritability
   Poor feeding
   Vomiting

7. *What is the classification of the patient's medication?*

   Tempra (acetaminophen)   — Analgesic

Chapter 22
Behavioural Disorders

Behaviour can be described as a patient's conduct and activities as observed by others. Society, religions, and gender constraints have a substantial impact on what is considered normal. They also define what may be considered abnormal. Presentations of abnormal behaviour may have a number of causes, including psychiatric issues, depression, anxiety disorder, substance use, or impulse disorders. Depression and suicide may also be linked to anxiety or impulse disorders. Through assessment, the paramedic should rule out potential medical causes of abnormal behaviour, such as diabetic-related emergencies or head trauma, before assuming that a behavioural emergency exists. Empathy and a non-judgmental approach are key to developing a rapport with patients, and scene safety is paramount.

CASE 22.1

At 16:00hrs, you are dispatched to 42 Paget Street North, New Liskeard, Ontario, for a possible hanging. Dispatch advises that a father came home and found his 16-year-old son hanging from a coat rack in his closet. The father, Mike, has taken his son down and is performing CPR when you arrive. As you survey the scene, you see Christopher lying on the floor of his bedroom naked, with belts tied to both lower legs. His father tells you that when his son did not answer his call, he went to his room and found him hanging from the coat rack by a housecoat tie with padding around his neck. You observe what looks to be semen on Christopher's chest and abdomen. Mike tells you that his son would have arrived home 30 minutes prior and was scheduled to go to a job interview at 17:00hrs. The father is extremely upset and questions why his son would have tried to kill himself: he was a good student and happy.

Initial Assessment Findings & Chief Complaint

LOA	Unconscious.
A	Patent.
B	Apneic.
C	VSA, no carotid pulses present.
Wet Check	Bodily fluids on chest and abdomen.
CC	Apparent hanging.

History

S	Patient is VSA with no obvious trauma noted.
A	Environmental.
M	Flovent, salbutamol, Tetracyn
P	Asthma.
L	Lunch at school.
E	The patient probably came home around 15:30hrs from school. He was found with padding and a housecoat tie around his neck, hanging from a coat rack in his closet. His legs and knees were touching the ground. The father cut him down, loosened the tie from his son's neck, called 911, and began CPR. CPR has been in progress for approximately five minutes.

Assessment

H/N	Face is cyanosed, with no ligature marks on his neck.
Chest	Unremarkable.
ABD	Unremarkable.
Back	Unremarkable.
Pelvis	Stable.
Ext	No obvious trauma, but lower extremities are more cyanosed than the rest of the body.

Vitals

BP	0
P	0
RR	0
Pupils	PERL 5 mm, non-reactive
GCS	1+1+1=3
BS	n/a
Pulse oximetry	0
Skin	Pale, cyanosed

Pain Assessment

O	n/a
P	n/a
Q	n/a
R	n/a
S	n/a
T	n/a

Cardiac Monitor

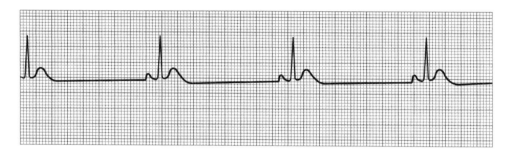

Figure 22.1

Initial Treatment Post Assessment

Initial assessment reveals that the patient is VSA. The airway should be patent, an OPA inserted, and CPR continued. The defibrillator should be attached as the patient is presenting in a non-shockable rhythm. Local protocol would dictate that CPR be continued throughout assessment and treatment. After two minutes of CPR, the patient's ECG should be reanalyzed if an SAED is being used. Other airway adjuncts such as a Combitube or LMA can be used to further secure the patient's airway. An ACP should intubate with an ETT no. 8 and confirm tube placement. An intravenous should be established and a 20 ml/kg fluid bolus initiated. Epinephrine 1.0 mg and/or atropine 1.0 mg should be administered via IV. CPR should continue, and if there is no change in the patient's rhythm or presentation, further doses of medication should be administered. The patient should be secured to the stretcher and transport to a hospital initiated.

En route, there is no change in the patient's condition, although there is a change in his ECG.

Cardiac Monitor

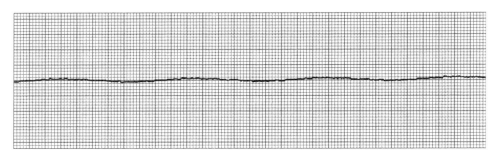

Figure 22.2

Treatment Continued

CPR and medication protocol should be continued en route to the hospital.

Differential Diagnosis

- Auto-erotic asphyxiation.

Test Your Knowledge

1. What was significant about the patient's positioning and the padding under the tie around his neck?
2. What is auto-erotic asphyxiation?
3. Was Christopher's death a suicide?
4. What was the actual cause of Christopher's death?
5. Why should Christopher not have a collar and board applied to stabilize his c-spine?
6. What classifications are the patient's medications?
7. What ECG is the patient presenting with?
8. What is difficult for the father and others affected by this incident?
9. What is this act of self-gratification commonly labelled by law-enforcement agencies?

CASE 22.2

You are dispatched to 48 17th Street West, Prince Albert, British Columbia, for an aggressive patient. You are met by the patient's sister Tracy, who tells you that Robert is acting weird. She says he can't sit still and is scaring her because he is uncontrollable, angry, and keeps yelling things that don't make sense. She says Robert is manic-depressive and just broke up with his girlfriend. He is 21 years old. She further reports that he is usually fine when he takes his medication, but she is afraid he stopped taking it some time ago. She wants to stay in the house, but cannot as long as he is there. She also wants him to go to the hospital, but he won't go. While you are talking to Tracy, two police cruisers arrive as Robert exits. He approaches the officers and begins struggling with them. After a few minutes, they are able to restrain him.

Initial Assessment Findings & Chief Complaint

LOA	Conscious, confused.
A	Patent.
B	Shallow but regular; appears to have alcohol on his breath.
C	Strong radial pulse.
Wet Check	Unremarkable.
CC	Erratic behaviour.

History

S	Patient is aggressive.
A	None.
M	carbamezapine, anafranil.
P	Bipolar disorder.
L	CNO.
E	The patient began bizarre behaviour a day or so earlier, is not making sense, and is aggressive toward people.

Assessment

H/N	Unremarkable.
Chest	Unremarkable, equal air entry bilaterally.
ABD	Soft/non-tender.
Back	Unremarkable.
Pelvis	Stable.
Ext	Equal strength and mobility.

Vitals

BP	140/92
P	150
RR	24 shallow
Pupils	PERL 4 mm
GCS	4+4+6=14
BS	5.1 mmol/l
Pulse oximetry	99%
Skin	Warm, diaphoretic

Pain Assessment

O	n/a
P	n/a
Q	n/a
R	n/a
S	n/a
T	n/a

Cardiac Monitor

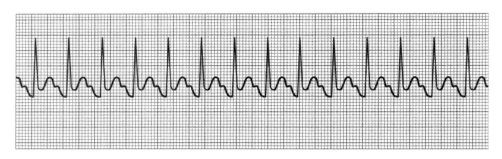

Figure 22.3

Initial Treatment Post Assessment

Although the patient has been restrained by police, a thorough assessment is still required and should be carried out. A complete set of vitals should be obtained, including SPO2 and blood glucometry to rule out hypoxia and hypo- or hyperglycemia. Cardiac monitoring should be initiated and oxygen administered, if accepted. An intravenous may be started. An ACP may administer Versed or other benzodiazepines if within local protocol.

En route to the hospital, the patient subsides and asks to have the restraints removed. His vital signs remain stable.

Treatment Continued

- The patient should remain restrained for the safety of the paramedics. Ongoing supportive care and assessment should continue.

Differential Diagnosis

- Bipolar disorder.

Test Your Knowledge

1. Why is the patient presenting with aggression and bizarre behaviour?
2. What best describes bipolar disorder or manic depression?
3. What are the classifications of the patient's medications?
4. What is the best approach for dealing with a bipolar patient?
5. What is the most important decision a paramedic can make when arriving on the scene of a patient in this state?
6. What other states can a bipolar patient present in?
7. What ECG is the patient presenting with?
8. En route to the hospital, what should a paramedic do to control the situation?

CASE 22.3

You are dispatched at 15:30hrs to the rear of 212 Green Street, Summerside, Prince Edward Island, for police assistance. On arrival, you notice several police cars with a group of officers standing behind one of them. One officer yells at you to come quickly, as there is a man who he thinks isn't breathing. He reports that police were called to a disturbance where a 34-year-old man with a long psychiatric history was acting in a bizarre fashion. The police officer tells you that two other officers were involved in a scuffle with the man, and it took all three of them to subdue him with night sticks. In the altercation, says the police officer, many punches were exchanged. They handcuffed the man, secured his legs to his hands behind him, and placed him on his stomach in the police van. Approximately eight minutes later, they noticed he wasn't breathing and called for EMS. Your time of arrival was two to three minutes later. The police begin to unlock the handcuffs.

Initial Assessment Findings & Chief Complaint

LOA	Unconscious.
A	Patent.
B	Apneic.
C	VSA.
Wet Check	Blood on hands.
CC	VSA after altercation with police.

History

S	VSA.
A	CNO.
M	Risperdal, Zyprexa.
P	Schizophrenia.
L	CNO.
E	The patient started acting bizarrely and had to be subdued by police with physical intervention. The patient's arms and legs were then tied and he was placed in the police van. He stopped breathing some time later, and EMS were called.

Assessment

H/N	Unremarkable, cyanosis in face.
Chest	Abrasions present on anterior chest.
ABD	Soft, unremarkable.
Back	Unremarkable.
Pelvis	Stable.
Ext	Abrasions on hands and track marks on left antecubital fossa.

Vitals

BP	0
P	0
RR	0
Pupils	PERL 5 mm, non-reactive
GCS	1+1+1=3
BS	5.0 mmol/l
Pulse oximetry	88% post resuscitation
Skin	Pale, cyanosed

Pain Assessment

O	n/a
P	n/a
Q	n/a
R	n/a
S	n/a
T	n/a

Cardiac Monitor

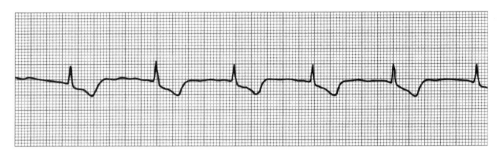

Figure 22.4

Initial Treatment Post Assessment

The patient should be turned on his back and ABCs assessed to confirm VSA. An OPA should be inserted and two-person CPR initiated immediately for two minutes. During this time, a defibrillator should be attached and an ECG interpreted at the conclusion of the CPR cycle. The PCP should continue the cycle as equipment is prepared for transport. An intermediate airway may also be utilized if available. An intravenous should be secured and a fluid bolus initiated. With the patient presenting in a PEA, an ACP should perform intubation and confirm appropriate placement of the ETT. Medications such as epinephrine and atropine should be administered intravenously according to local protocol. CPR should continue on scene and en route to the hospital. An ACP should continue the drug routine en route.

Three minutes after your arrival, the patient regains a weak carotid pulse that begins to strengthen. He is still apneic.

Cardiac Monitor

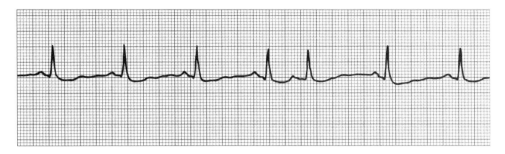

Figure 22.5

Treatment Continued

The patient should be transported promptly and ventilated via a BVM. The fluid bolus should be continued until a complete set of vitals are obtained, including SPO2, blood glucometry, and an adequate blood pressure. The patient should be monitored en route.

Differential Diagnosis

- Possible agitated delirium.
- Positional asphyxia.
- Possible drug-induced psychosis.

Test Your Knowledge

1. What is significant about the patient's position when you arrive on scene?
2. What may be the cause of the patient's progression to VSA?
3. What is agitated delirium?
4. What is schizophrenia?
5. Should hog-tying be utilized in the field for patient restraint?
6. What are the classifications of the patient's medications?
7. What are signs and symptoms of schizophrenia?
8. What ECG is the patient presenting with on arrival and post-resuscitation?

Answers
Case 22.1

1. ***What was significant about the patient's positioning and the padding under the tie around his neck?***
   A survey of the scene and the recognition of the protective pad around the patient's neck make it clear that death was not intended. A patient intent on suicide does not typically utilize padding to cushion their neck. Also, the presence of semen on the patient indicates a solo sexual activity.

2. *What is auto-erotic asphyxiation?*

    Auto-erotic asphyxiation, also known as sexual hanging, is an abnormal sexual behaviour. It is the practice of inducing cerebral anoxia while masturbating to orgasm. It is thought that hanging physiologically enhances orgasm as it interferes with blood supply to the brain. Forms of asphyxiation in this kind of auto-eroticism include placing a plastic bag over the head or inhaling aerosols.

3. *Was Christopher's death a suicide?*

    Based on Christopher's presentation and the father's description of his demeanor, this is not considered a suicide; it is an auto-erotic asphyxiation. The state of anoxia, once reached, weakens the patient's judgment and control over his body. An accidental death can result from the failure of the patient to follow through on his self-rescue plan. This appears to be what happened in this case since Christopher was kneeling on the ground; all he would have had to do to live was stand up.

4. *What was the actual cause of Christopher's death?*

    The actual cause of death was anoxia from asphyxiation.

5. *Why should Christopher not have a collar and board applied to stabilize his c-spine?*

    The mechanism of injury dictates that the cause of the VSA was not trauma but strangulation or anoxia; therefore, spinal immobilization is not warranted.

6. *What classifications are the patient's medications?*

Flovent (fluticasone propionate)	– Corticosteroid
salbutamol (Ventolin)	– Selective beta2-adrenergic bronchodilator
Tetracyn (tetracycline)	– Broad-spectrum antibiotic

7. *What ECG is the patient presenting with?*

    The patient was originally presenting in a pulseless electrical activity (PEA) and progressed to asystole.

8. *What is difficult for the father and others affected by this incident?*

    Families and survivors are often puzzled by what seems to be bizarre behaviour. They are left struggling not only with the grief and guilt of a sudden tragedy, but often with embarrassing questions regarding auto-erotic asphyxiation. As with suicide, there are many unanswered questions, and Christopher is not around to explain what his intentions were.

9. *What is this act of self-gratification commonly labelled by law-enforcement agencies?*

    Auto-erotic asphyxiation is sometimes labelled or misrepresented as suicide or homicide. When a victim is found, embarrassed family members may attempt to clean bodily fluids from the patient. Once the fluids are removed, the correlation between death and sexual gratification has been eliminated. Without such evidence, law-enforcement agencies may conclude that the death was a suicide.

Case 22.2

1. *Why is the patient presenting with aggression and bizarre behaviour?*

    The patient is probably presenting this way because he has stopped taking his medications. Bipolar patients will not have severe fluctuations of emotion if there is compliance in taking medication.

2. *What best describes bipolar disorder or manic depression?*

    Bipolar depression is described as occurrences of mania cycling with occurrences of depression. Manic episodes usually escalate over several days, with a period of elevated and irritable moods. The patient may also present with hostility and racing thoughts and become argumentative, sarcastic, and sometimes violent, especially when plans are thwarted. This is usually followed by a depressive and sometimes vegetative state.

3. *What are the classifications of the patient's medications?*

carbamezapine (Tegretol)	– Anti-convulsant
Anafranil (clomipramine)	– Antidepressant

4. **What is the best approach for dealing with a bipolar patient?**

   The best approach to dealing with a bipolar patient, regardless of the patient's state, is to maintain a calm, protective, and non-confrontational demeanor.

5. **What is the most important decision a paramedic can make when arriving on the scene of a patient in this state?**

   The most important decision a paramedic should make is the decision of whether or not it is safe to approach the patient. This information can usually be obtained from family members or others who may be involved with the patient. Many patients are reluctant to accept medical attention at varying aspects of their cycle.

6. **What other states can a bipolar patient present in?**

   A bipolar patient can also present in a depressive state, with loss of interest, feelings of worthlessness, and suicidal thoughts. Delusions and hallucinations can occur in both manic and depressive stages.

7. **What ECG is the patient presenting with?**

   The patient is presenting in a sinus tachycardia.

8. **En route to the hospital, what should a paramedic do to control the situation?**

   En route to the hospital, the paramedic should maintain a non-threatening demeanor with a calm, supportive approach to patient care.

Case 22.3

1. **What is significant about the patient's position when you arrive on scene?**

   The patient is positioned face down and hog-tied. This is a significant finding, since the position may have contributed to the patient's state.

2. **What may have contributed to the patient's progression to VSA?**

   The following factors may have contributed to a VSA state:

   Hog-tied positioning
   Agitated delirium
   Overdose of street drugs

3. **What is agitated delirium?**

   Agitated delirium is characterized by a severe disturbance in the level of consciousness and a change in mental status over a relatively short period of time, usually manifested in mental and physiological arousal, agitation, hostility, and heightened sympathetic stimulation.

4. **What is schizophrenia?**

   Schizophrenia is characterized by impairments in the perception of reality and a dysfunctional relationship with society. Patients typically demonstrate disorganized thinking, such as delusions or hallucinations.

5. **Should hog-tying be utilized in the field for patient restraint?**

   There is substantial evidence that hog-tying or using hobble restraints may create or contribute to a condition called restraint asphyxia. This position clearly affects breathing in situations requiring high oxygen demand, since it impairs chest-wall and diaphragmatic movement. Hyperactivity, compounded by a patient's struggles, contribute to apnea. Although there is limited evidence regarding the position alone, research suggests that together with contributing factors such as illicit drug ingestion, hyperthermia, hyperactivity, and catecholamine stimulation, hog-typing compounds breathing problems and increases the chances of asphyxia.

6. *What are the classifications of the patient's medications?*

   Risperdal (risperidone) – Antipsychotic
   Zyprexa (olanzapine) – Antipsychotic

7. *What are signs and symptoms of schizophrenia?*

   The following behaviours are signs and symptoms of schizophrenia:

   Withdrawal from activities and social contacts
   Irrational, angry, or fearful responses to friends and family
   Deterioration in studies or work
   Inappropriate use of language, words that do not make sense
   Deterioration in personal hygiene
   Hearing voices or sounds others don't hear
   Seeing people or things others don't see
   Occasional acts of violence

8. *What ECG is the patient presenting with on arrival and post-resuscitation?*

   The patient was presenting in a PEA and progressed to an NSR with PAC post-resuscitation.

Chapter 23
Gynecology

Other than labour and delivery, the most common emergencies involving women of childbearing age are abdominal pain and vaginal bleeding. For women in this group, abdominal pain is often connected with the reproductive organs. Many patient presentations can pose a life threat, so a thorough assessment should be completed. In addition to typical medical history questions, specific details regarding sexual activity and the possibility of pregnancy must be obtained. Although asking such questions will sometimes be uncomfortable, it may help in obtaining a differential diagnosis.

CASE 23.1

You are dispatched at 13:25hrs to Central Suites Hotel, Yellowknife, for a 27-year-old female patient with abdominal pain. She greets you at the hotel room door. She says her name is Samyia and that she has had sharp lower abdominal pain for the past 45 minutes. Her pain is centralized to the RLQ. She appears pale and diaphoretic and is obviously uncomfortable with the pain. She explains that she is from Yellowknife but now lives in Stewart, British Columbia, and is home for a few days for a wedding.

Initial Assessment Findings & Chief Complaint

LOA	Conscious and alert.
A	Patent.
B	Shallow but regular.
C	Strong radial pulses present.
Wet Check	Unremarkable.
CC	RLQ pain.

History

S	Sharp RLQ pain.
A	None.
M	Robaxisal, Advil.
P	Back strain two weeks earlier; taking medication for it.
L	Lunch.
E	Had generalized pain in the abdomen this morning, which has increased in severity and is now in the RLQ.

Assessment

H/N	Unremarkable, no JVD, trachea midline.
Chest	Unremarkable, equal air entry.
ABD	Diffuse tenderness on palpation to the RLQ.
Back	Unremarkable.
Pelvis	Stable.
Ext	Equal strength and mobility.

Vitals

BP	108/68
P	75, strong and regular
RR	16
Pupils	PERL 3+ mm
GCS	4+5+6=15
BS	n/a
Pulse oximetry	99%
Skin	Pale, diaphoretic

Pain Assessment

O	Gradual
P	While at rest
Q	Sharp
R	None
S	8/10
T	45 minutes

Cardiac Monitor

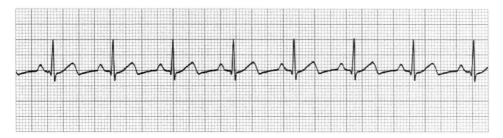

Figure 23.1

Initial Treatment Post Assessment

The patient should be assessed and a complete set of vitals obtained. An ECG interpretation should also be completed. Oxygen should be administered via a high concentration mask. A complete obstetrical history should be obtained from the patient, including the date of her last menstrual cycle, in order to explore the possibility of pregnancy-related complications. The patient says she is sexually active and had a slight one-day period the previous month, which was unusual for her. An intravenous should be initiated and infused at TKVO. There is no additional treatment that an ACP can render.

En route to the hospital, the patient becomes more lethargic and complains of increased tenderness in her abdomen. She also says her shoulder is now hurting. Her vitals are BP 88/68, P 150, and RR 16, and her skin is pale and diaphoretic. She tells you she is having vaginal bleeding, and you see that her pants are saturated at the front.

Cardiac Monitor

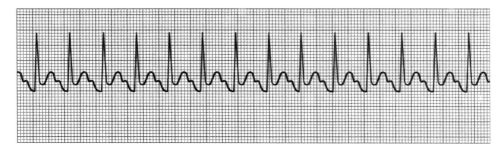

Figure 23.2

Treatment Continued

The intravenous rate should be increased to deliver a 20 ml/kg bolus. Abdominal pads should be used to absorb vaginal bleeding. Rapid transport to an emergency department should continue.

Differential Diagnosis

- Ruptured ectopic pregnancy.

Test Your Knowledge

1. What are the predisposing factors for ectopic pregnancy?
2. Where do the majority of ectopic pregnancies occur?
3. What is the patient's ECG interpretation?
4. Depending on the amount of intra-abdominal bleeding, where might the patient have referred pain?
5. Why is questioning a patient regarding the possibility of pregnancy appropriate in all female assessments?
6. What is the patient at risk of, if an ectopic pregnancy is not diagnosed and treated early?
7. What classifications are the patient's medications?

CASE 23.2

You are dispatched to a train station in Sipiwesk, Manitoba, at 14:30hrs for a female patient with abdominal pain. On arrival, you meet a 19-year-old girl shuffling toward a nearby bench. She looks unwell and appears pale. She introduces herself as Tracie and explains that she has had pain before but never this bad. She tells you it has been awful for the last day but that she is on her way home to New Brunswick and thought she would be okay.

Initial Assessment Findings & Chief Complaint

LOA	Conscious and alert.
A	Patent.
B	Shallow but regular.
C	Strong radial pulses.
Wet Check	Unremarkable.
CC	Lower abdominal pain.

History

S	Patient complains of lower abdominal pain, vaginal discharge, and chills.
A	Penicillin.
M	Birth control pills.
P	None.
L	Ate on the train.
E	The patient has been complaining of diffuse pain in the lower abdomen that increased in severity approximately 45 minutes ago, making it difficult for her to walk. She tells you she has had vaginal discharge today and some minimal bleeding, and is midway through her cycle.

Assessment

H/N	No JVD, trachea midline.
Chest	Unremarkable, with equal air entry bilaterally.
ABD	Complains of lower abdominal pain that worsens with movement. On palpation, the pain increases with rebound tenderness.
Back	Unremarkable.
Pelvis	Stable.
Ext	Equal strength and mobility with strong peripheral pulses.

Vitals

BP	108/68
P	75, regular
RR	18
Pupils	PERL 3+ mm
GCS	4+5+6=15
BS	n/a
Pulse oximetry	98%
Skin	Pale, ill-looking

Pain Assessment

O	2 days
P	Occurred while at rest
Q	Sharp
R	No radiation
S	10/10
T	Episode lasted approximately 45 minutes.

Cardiac Monitor

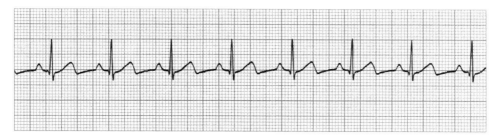

Figure 23.3

Initial Treatment Post Assessment

An initial assessment should be performed on the patient and vitals obtained. A cardiac monitor should be applied and an ECG interpreted. Oxygen should be administered via a nasal cannula at 4–6 lpm. The patient should be transported in a position of comfort, possibly in a knee to chest position. An intravenous should be initiated and run at TKVO. ACPs follow the same protocol of treatment. The patient should be questioned regarding the possibility of pregnancy.

En route to the hospital, the patient says she had her normal cycle the previous month but started having mild bleeding and discharge today. She tells you she is sexually active, is on the birth control pill, and is not pregnant.

Treatment Continued

Further treatment should involve ongoing assessment of vitals and transportation to the nearest hospital. The intravenous should continue at TKVO.

Differential Diagnosis

- Pelvic Inflammatory Disease (PID).

Test Your Knowledge

1. What is pelvic inflammatory disease (PID)?
2. What are the most common causes of PID?
3. What are the predisposing factors for PID?
4. What are the typical signs/symptoms of PID?
5. Why is the patient more comfortable in a knees-to-chest position during transport?
6. What ECG is the patient presenting with?
7. What can PID lead to if not diagnosed and treated?

Answers

Case 23.1

1. *What are the predisposing factors for ectopic pregnancy?*

    Predisposing factors for ectopic pregnancy can include:

    Pelvic inflammatory disease
    Previous ectopic pregnancies
    Tubal surgery
    Use of IUD
    Tubal pathology

2. *Where do the majority of ectopic pregnancies occur?*

    The majority of ectopic pregnancies occur in the fallopian tube. Ectopic pregnancies can also occur in the abdominal cavity.

3. *What is the patient's ECG interpretation?*

    The patient is presenting in a normal sinus rhythm and progresses to a sinus tachycardia.

4. *Depending on the amount of intra-abdominal bleeding, where might the patient have referred pain?*

    The patient might have referred pain in the shoulder.

5. *Why is questioning a patient regarding the possibility of pregnancy appropriate in all female assessments?*

    All patients of child-bearing age should be asked whether they are sexually active and if there is a possibility of pregnancy. Asking the patient the date of her last menstrual cycle is important in order to determine the possibility of a gynecological emergency.

6. *What is the patient at risk of, if an ectopic pregnancy is not diagnosed and treated early?*

    The patient is at risk of hypovolemia if the ectopic pregnancy is not diagnosed.

7. **What classifications are the patient's medications?**

   Robaxisal (methocarbamol and ASA) — Skeletal muscle relaxant
   Advil (ibuprofen) — NSAID

Case 23.2

1. **What is pelvic inflammatory disease (PID)?**

   Pelvic inflammatory disease is an infection of the female reproductive organs caused by bacteria, fungus, or a virus.

2. **What are the most common causes of PID?**

   The most common causes of PID are chlamydia (Chlamydia trachmatis) or gonorrhea (Neisseria gonorrhoeae). These infections can sometimes go undetected until the presentation of PID.

3. **What are the predisposing factors for PID?**

   The predisposing factors for PID include:

   Multiple sexual partners
   Use of an IUD
   Recent gynecological procedures

4. **What are the typical signs and symptoms of PID?**

   The typical signs and symptoms of PID include:

   Ill appearance
   Fever or chills
   Nausea
   Vomiting
   Foul smelling vaginal discharge
   Mid-cycle bleeding
   Diffuse abdominal pain with rebound tenderness
   Asymptomatic (no symptoms)

5. **Why is the patient more comfortable in a knees-to-chest position during transport?**

   The patient is more comfortable in a knees-to-chest position as it decreases tension on the perineum.

6. **What ECG is the patient presenting with?**

   The patient is presenting in a normal sinus rhythm.

7. **What can PID lead to if not diagnosed and treated?**

   The infection and inflammation of PID can lead to scarring and adhesions on the fallopian tubal lumens.

Chapter 24
Obstetrics

Childbirth is a normal process and obstetrical emergencies are relatively uncommon. In most cases, patients are under the care of an obstetrician, potential complications are discovered early, and the patient follows a treatment plan throughout pregnancy. Still, paramedics must be aware of potential complications and how to intervene for a successful delivery. Complications arise when dealing with more than one patient in any situation that may not be routine. Effective communication with the mother and control of the baby's birth will promote success in obstetric emergencies.

CASE 24.1

You are dispatched to 117 Toronto Avenue, Wawa, Ontario, for a possible childbirth. Dispatch advises that the patient is 22 years old and that this is her second pregnancy. They advise that the patient's contractions are approximately two minutes apart and are lasting for one minute. As you arrive at the residence, you find an anxious couple awaiting your arrival. Natasha is lying on the couch covered with a sheet from the bed. Her husband explains that her water broke the previous night and they thought the baby might come soon. They wanted to have a home birth. Natasha says she has a splitting headache and that her vision has been blurry for the past two days. She is tired and just wants to have the baby and rest.

Initial Assessment Findings & Chief Complaint

LOA	Conscious and alert.
A	Patent.
B	Full volume.
C	Strong radial pulses.
Wet Check	Unremarkable.
CC	Expected childbirth.

History

S	Patient is complaining of contractions lasting for approximately one minute as well as a very severe frontal headache with blurred vision.
A	Latex.
M	enalapril, spronolactone, chlorpropamide.
P	Type 2 diabetes, PIH.
L	Breakfast.
E	Patient says the contractions are one minute apart and starting to occur more frequently. Her water broke the previous night, and she says her lower back is starting to hurt. She can barely lift her head from the pillow because of the severity of her headache.

Assessment

H/N	Unremarkable.
Chest	Equal air entry without adventitious sounds.
ABD	Soft/non-tender, uterus at costal margin.
Back	Unremarkable.
Pelvis	Stable.
Ext	Equal strength and mobility in extremities.

Vitals

BP	168/108
P	150, regular
RR	18 full volume
Pupils	PERL 3+ mm
GCS	4+5+6=15
BS	6.8 mmol/l
Pulse oximetry	98%
Skin	Normal, diaphoretic

Pain Assessment

O	n/a
P	n/a
Q	n/a
R	n/a
S	n/a
T	n/a

Cardiac Monitor

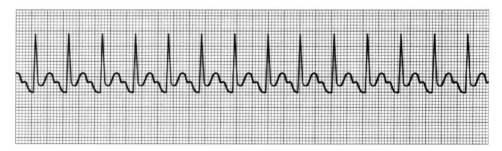

Figure 24.1

Initial Treatment Post Assessment

An appropriate obstetrical history should be determined while a physical assessment is performed. Vital signs and an ECG should be obtained from the patient. An inspection of the peritoneum should be completed to observe if any crowning is present and whether delivery is evident. The patient should be positioned on a stretcher as comfortably as possible, with a wedge under her left side. Oxygen via a high concentration mask should be administered.

En route to the hospital, Natasha tells you that she feels she has to push. Before you have the opportunity to undo the seatbelts and assess the peritoneum, you see Natasha pushing with the current contraction. As you uncover her, you see the baby's head being delivered.

Treatment Continued

Supporting the infant's head, instruct the mother to pant to allow you time to assess for a nuchal cord. Suction the baby's mouth and nose, if secretions are excessive. If the umbilical cord is not wrapped around the infant's neck, instruct the mother to push with the next contraction. Maintain support on the infant's head and neck with one hand, and use the other to assist and guide the delivery. Apply gentle pressure downward to deliver the anterior shoulder, and then upward to deliver the posterior shoulder. Once the infant has been delivered, suction the mouth and then the nose. Dry the baby to stimulate respirations and crying. Provide oxygen to an acrocyanotic infant via a blow-by tube at 6–8 lpm. Assess the infant's APGAR.

The infant is squirming actively, has a strong cry, is breathing at approximately RR 40, is pink with blue extremities, and has a heart rate of 130.

Treatment Continued

Continuously assess the infant and mother en route to the hospital. Assess the umbilical cord for absence of pulsations and apply clamps in two places, one approximately 15 cm from the infant's abdomen and another 5–7 cm further away. Cut the cord, have the mother hold the baby, and advise her to nurse if she desires.

Differential Diagnosis

- Childbirth.
- Pre-eclampsia.

Test Your Knowledge

1. When is it appropriate to cut an umbilical cord that is wrapped around a baby's neck?
2. What is a baby's APGAR?
3. What are the typical signs and symptoms of pre-eclampsia?
4. What classifications are the patient's medications?
5. What are risk factors for pre-eclampsia?
6. Natasha tells you that her due date is July 16th. How can you verify this?
7. What is a typical term pregnancy?
8. Besides PARA and GRAVIDA, what is another mnemonic that can help in the assessment of a pregnant patient?

CASE 24.2

At 03:20hrs, you are dispatched to 13 39th Street, Ponoka, Alberta, for a possible delivery. Dispatch advises that the call came from a frantic 28-year-old woman who is having a baby. The woman is alone in her bedroom and the front door is locked. She says her water has broken and contractions are regular and approximately 30 seconds apart. She also says she sees one foot outside her vagina. Dispatch is sending fire and police to the scene to assist with gaining entry. On arrival, you gain access and enter the bedroom, where the patient, Ashley, is lying supine on her bed. She appears very anxious and is pale and diaphoretic. As you approach and assess her, you see that she is experiencing a breech delivery with both feet protruding from her vagina.

Initial Assessment Findings & Chief Complaint

LOA	Conscious and alert.
A	Patent.
B	Regular at 20.
C	Weak radial pulses.
Wet Check	Bed is wet where the patient's water has broken.
CC	Patient is having contractions and is presenting with a breech delivery.

History

S	Patient complains of contractions relatively frequently, approximately every 30 seconds, lasting for one minute.
A	Environmental.
M	Diclectin.
P	Hyperemesis gravidarum.
L	Supper.
E	Patient went to bed with mild, infrequent contractions. At approximately midnight, her water broke and her contractions became more frequent and regular.

Assessment

H/N	Unremarkable.
Chest	Equal air entry bilaterally.
ABD	Soft/non-tender.
Back	Unremarkable.
Pelvis	Stable.
Ext	Unremarkable.

Vitals   Pain Assessment

BP	86/60	O	n/a
P	150, regular	P	n/a
RR	20	Q	n/a
Pupils	PERL 3+ mm	R	n/a
GCS	4+5+6=15	S	n/a
BS	n/a	T	n/a
Pulse oximetry	98%		
Skin	Pale, diaphoretic		

Cardiac Monitor

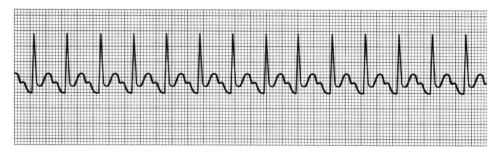

Figure 24.2

Initial Treatment Post Assessment

Initial treatment should include a thorough assessment, including vitals and an ECG interpretation. Oxygen via a high concentration mask should be administered. The patient should pant through contractions until the assessment is complete. Position the mother with her hips tilted and the right hip elevated. On her next contraction, have the patient push at will, allowing delivery while supporting the infant's legs and body as it arrives. When the umbilical cord is visible, check for a cord pulse. If the pulse is weak or absent, reposition the mother or elevate the infant's body to try to regain or strengthen the pulse. When the nape of the neck is visible, gently lift the infant's legs, avoiding hyperextension. Allow the head to deliver spontaneously. There is no significant treatment difference between a PCP or an ACP. An intravenous can be initiated and run at a conservative 20 ml/kg bolus.

You assess the umbilical cord pulse to be strong and regular. Three minutes later, the head has still not delivered. The patient is becoming more anxious and scared. There is still a strong cord pulse.

Treatment Continued

Slide your free hand into the lower end of the vagina and create a V shape on either side of the infant's mouth and nose. Push away from the infant's face, creating an opening for the child's airway. Slide the other hand into the upper end of the vagina over the infant's occiput and apply gentle downward pressure.

The head of the baby is now delivered and the infant is crying, exhibiting spontaneous respirations, and is peripherally cyanosed. The infant has a strong pulse of approximately 140.

Treatment Continued

Assess the infant's airway and suction the mouth and nose as required. After the umbilical cord stops pulsating, clamp and cut it. Allow the baby to nurse and begin transport to a hospital as soon as possible. Monitor the mother's and infant's vitals en route. The intravenous should be adjusted to run at TKVO.

Differential Diagnosis

- Breech delivery.

Test Your Knowledge

1. What is significant about the patient's position when you arrive on scene?
2. What ECG is the patient presenting with?
3. What is the classification of the patient's medication?
4. What is hyperemesis gravidarum?
5. The patient appears anxious with the circumstances, so what would explain her low blood pressure?
6. What is the appropriate treatment for the patient's hypotensive state?
7. If the infant is not delivered after gentle pressure is applied to the occiput, what is the next step?
8. After delivery, the infant is presenting with cyanosis in the extremities. What is another name for this condition?

CASE 24.3

You are dispatched to 127 Avenue de L'Abbe-Bourg, Chandler, Quebec, for a 35-year-old woman with acute abdominal pain and vaginal bleeding. Dispatch advises that the patient is in her 30th week of gestation with her first child. On arrival, the patient greets you at the door and tells you that she feels as if the baby is being ripped from inside her. She sits on a chair beside the door in obvious distress. She tells you her name is Marie Louise and that the baby is not due for another 10 weeks. She also says she has saturated two pads with blood in the hour since the pain started.

Initial Assessment Findings & Chief Complaint

LOA	Conscious and alert.
A	Patent.
B	Full volume at approximately RR 20.
C	Strong radial pulses.
Wet Check	Minimal vaginal bleeding.
CC	Tearing pain in her abdomen with mild vaginal bleeding.

History

S	Patient complaining of a sharp tearing feeling in her abdomen and vaginal bleeding.
A	None.
M	Lipitor, Synthroid, Xanax, ASA, Imitrex.
P	30 weeks gestation, thyroid disorder, anxiety, migraine headaches.
L	Normal meals.
E	The patient states that she had a sudden onset of sharp, tearing pain in her abdomen starting approximately one hour earlier. It has not subsided. She thought it would go away but after an hour she decided to call EMS. Her pregnancy has been normal thus far, and her last checkup at her obstetrician's office was okay. She also tells you that she had a tumble down a few stairs this morning, landing on her abdomen. She felt fine afterward and was not overly concerned.

Assessment

H/N	Unremarkable, no JVD, trachea midline.
Chest	Equal air entry bilaterally.
ABD	Stiff, board-like abdomen and no increased pain on palpation, but guarding is present.
Back	Unremarkable.
Pelvis	Stable.
Ext	Equal strength and mobility.

Vitals

BP	110/70
P	74
RR	20 shallow
Pupils	PERL 4+ mm
GCS	4+5+6=15
BS	n/a
Pulse oximetry	99%
Skin	Warm, diaphoretic

Pain Assessment

O	n/a
P	n/a
Q	n/a
R	n/a
S	n/a
T	n/a

Cardiac Monitor

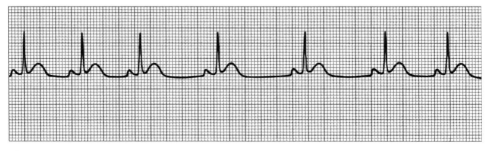

Figure 24.3

Initial Treatment Post Assessment

The patient should be assessed and c-spine ruled out due to the fall. A complete set of vitals should be obtained, including an ECG interpretation. Further obstetrical history should be obtained from the patient. Oxygen should be administered via a high concentration mask at 12 lpm. An assessment of the vaginal area should be completed in order to evaluate the cessation or continuation of vaginal bleeding. An intravenous should be initiated and run at TKVO, and the patient should be transported in a left lateral recumbent position on the stretcher to the ambulance and then the hospital.

En route to the hospital, the patient complains of increased pain and increased vaginal bleeding. Her vitals are BP 90/50, P 100 in sinus tachycardia, RR 22 and shallow with a SPO2 of 98%, and paler skin with increased diaphoresis.

Treatment Continued

The intravenous should be opened to run at a bolus of 20 ml/kg to sustain a BP of 100/P. Additional sanitary napkins or abdominal pads should be utilized to absorb the additional vaginal bleeding. A further update of the patient's condition should be relayed to the receiving obstetrical unit of the hospital.

Differential Diagnosis

- Abruptio placentae.

Test Your Knowledge

1. What are possible causes of abruptio placentae?
2. What are the classifications of the patient's medications?
3. What ECG is the patient presenting with?
4. Is abruptio placentae a life-threatening condition?
5. Is external bleeding always evident with the presentation of abruptio placentae?
6. How do signs and symptoms of abruptio placentae vary depending on the location of the abruption?
7. What could have caused the abruptio placentae in your patient?

Answers

Case 24.1

1. ***When is it appropriate to cut an umbilical cord that is wrapped around a baby's neck?***
   If an umbilical cord is loosely wrapped around a baby's neck, an attempt should be made to slip it over the baby's head. If the cord is wrapped more than once or is too tight to remove, two clamps should be placed 5-7 cm apart and the cord cut. It can then be removed safely from around the baby's neck.

2. **What is a baby's APGAR?**

   APGAR is a quick method for evaluating the clinical status of a newborn. It is usually assessed at the one- and five-minute mark. A score of 0 through 2 is assigned for each category: appearance, pulse, grimace, activity and respiration.

   A: 1
   P: 2
   G: 2
   A: 2
   R: 2
   Total: 9

3. **What are the typical signs and symptoms of pre-eclampsia?**

   The classic signs of pre-eclampsia include:

   Generalized edema in face, hands, and feet
   BP > 140/90 (severe eclampsia if diastolic BP is greater than 110)
   Proteinuria

4. **What classifications are the patient's medications?**

   enalapril (Vasotec) — ACE Inhibiter
   spironolactone (Aldactone) — Potassium-sparing diuretic
   chlorpropamide (Diabenese) — Oral blood-glucose-lowering agent

5. **What are risk factors of pre-eclampsia?**

   The risk factors of pre-eclampsia include:

   Excessive amniotic fluid
   First pregnancy
   Pre-existing hypertension
   Multiple gestations

6. **Natasha tells you that her due date is July 16th. How can you verify this?**

   You can verify the due date by knowing the date of the first day of Natasha's last menstrual cycle. With this information, Nagel's rule can be used to calculate and verify the due date.

   Date (of last menstrual period) − 3 months + 7 days = due date

7. **What is a typical term pregnancy?**

   Normal pregnancy consists of 280 days or 40 weeks. Term pregnancy consists of the period between 37 and 40 weeks.

8. **Besides PARA and GRAVIDA, what is another mnemonic that can help in the assessment of a pregnant patient?**

   The mnemonic GTPAL can be used in the assessment of a pregnant patient.

   G = Gravida (number of pregnancies)
   T = Term babies (number brought to term, i.e., after 37 weeks)
   P = Premature (number of children born before 37 weeks)
   A = Abortions (number of spontaneous or therapeutic abortions)
   L = Living children (number currently living)

9. **What ECG is the patient presenting in?**

   The patient is presenting in a sinus tachycardia.

Case 24.2

1. **What is significant about the patient's position when you arrive on scene?**

   The patient is positioned supine with the infant's legs exiting the vagina in anticipation of delivery. The mother's legs should be repositioned and flexed, creating a larger potential opening to aid in delivery.

2. **What ECG is the patient presenting with?**

   The patient is presenting with a sinus tachycardia.

3. **What is the classification of the patient's medication?**

   Diclectin (doxylamine succinate with pyridoxine HCl) – Anti-nauseant for pregnancy

4. **What is hyperemesis gravidarum?**

   Hyperemesis gravidarum is a rare complication in pregnancy causing unrelenting, excessive pregnancy-related nausea or vomiting that prevents adequate intake of food and/or fluids.

5. **The patient appears anxious with the circumstances, so what would explain her low blood pressure?**

   The patient does not appear to have a significant amount of external bleeding, so her hypotensive state may be caused by supine-hypotensive or vena cava syndrome. This occurs when the uterus compresses the inferior vena cava while the mother is lying in a supine position.

6. **What is the appropriate treatment for the patient's hypotensive state?**

   A fluid bolus should be initiated and the mother moved to a gradual left lateral recumbent position.

7. **If the infant is not delivered after gentle pressure is applied to the occiput, what is the next step?**

   If the infant is still not delivered after applying gentle pressure to the occiput, place your free hand (the hand not maintaining the airway opening) slightly above the maternal symphysis pubis and apply firm downward pressure with the heel.

8. **After delivery, the infant is presenting with cyanosis in the extremities. What is another name for this condition?**

   Peripheral cyanosis, also called acrocyanosis, is very common after delivery. If an infant does not respond well, stimulation should resolve this condition (e.g., vigorous drying, flicking the soles of the feet, and rubbing the child's back).

Case 24.3

1. **What are possible causes of abruptio placentae?**

   The possible causes of abruptio placenta include:

   Trauma
   Maternal hypertension
   Multiparity
   Increased maternal age
   Previous abruptions

2. **What are the classifications of the patient's medications?**

Lipitor (atorvastatin calcium)	– Lipid-lowering agent
Synthroid (levothyroxine)	– Supplemental hypothyroidism therapy
Xanax (alprazolam)	– Benzodiazepine
ASA (acetylsalicylic acid)	– Anti-inflammatory analgesic
Imitrex (sumatriptan succinate)	– Migraine headache therapy

3. **What ECG is the patient presenting with?**

   The patient is presenting in a sinus dysrhythmia.

4. *Is abruptio placentae a life-threatening condition?*

   Abruptio placenta is a life-threatening obstetrical emergency. Immediate recognition and intervention is imperative to maintain maternal oxygenation and perfusion. Rapid transport to an emergency facility with neonatal care is imperative.

5. *Is external bleeding always evident with the presentation of abruptio placentae?*

   Bleeding is not always evident with abruptio placentae. It is dependent on the location and character of the abruption in the uterus.

6. *How do signs and symptoms of abruptio placentae vary depending on the location of the abruption?*

   Partial abruptions can be marginal or central. In central abruption, the placenta separates centrally, and bleeding is trapped between the placenta and the uterine wall. The patient would present with sharp tearing pain and minimal or no bleeding. Marginal abruptions present with bleeding but no pain, as there is no pressure built up on the nerve endings within the uterus and as blood is not trapped. With complete abruptio placentae, there is substantial blood loss and hypotension.

7. *What could have caused the abruptio placentae in your patient?*

   The patient told you that she had a fall earlier in the day and landed on her abdomen. Placental separation can occasionally occur within hours of an acceleration or deceleration injury even though there may be no evidence of abdominal trauma on your assessment. Blunt minor trauma that does not involve acceleration or deceleration usually does not cause fetal injury because of the presence of amniotic fluid.

Division 3 Other Emergencies

Chapter 25
Neonatology

Once babies are born, they progress and grow through normal stages of development. The term "neonate" refers to a child at the developmental stage from birth to one month old. Neonates should be treated using the same priorities that apply to all patients. The vast majority of newborns require no special care beyond airway suctioning, stimulation, and maintenance of body temperature. In the case of a neonate requiring intervention, however, the promptness of the paramedic's decisions and intervention will make a significant difference in the outcome of the emergency.

CASE 25.1

At 11:30hrs, you are dispatched to 42 Canterbury Drive, Osoyoos, British Columbia, for a distressed infant. On arrival you are greeted by a woman, Kim Soo, and rushed into the house where Kim Soo's mother is holding her one-month-old grandson. As you approach, you observe that the infant is cyanosed and appears dyspneic. The mother tells you that the grandmother was feeding the baby when he began to turn dark blue and have trouble breathing. She thought he had choked on milk, so she burped him, but nothing changed.

Initial Assessment Findings & Chief Complaint

LOA	Conscious/restless.
A	Patent.
B	Laboured.
C	Strong brachial pulse.
Wet Check	Unremarkable.
CC	Dyspnea.

History

S	Dyspnea with cyanosis.
A	None.
M	Amoxil.
P	Healthy, current ear infection.
L	Currently.
E	The patient was feeding and had a sudden onset of hyperpnea and cyanosis.

Assessment

H/N	Cyanosed face, no JVD, trachea midline.
Chest	Accessory muscle usage, but air entry is equal and bilateral.
ABD	Soft/non-tender.
Back	Unremarkable.
Pelvis	Stable.
Ext	Excessive movement of upper and lower extremities with cyanosis.

Vitals & Pain Assessment

BP	80/60	O	n/a
P	130	P	n/a
RR	50	Q	n/a
Pupils	PERL 4+ mm	R	n/a
GCS	4+5+6=15	S	n/a
BS	n/a	T	n/a
Pulse oximetry	88%		
Skin	Cyanosed		

Cardiac Monitor

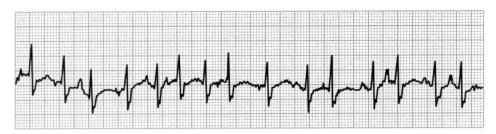

Figure 25.1

Initial Treatment Post Assessment

The child should be assessed and his vitals obtained, including SPO2. The patient should receive high concentrations of oxygen via a non-rebreather mask or blow-by tube. Cardiac monitoring should be performed and rapid transport initiated. Ongoing re-evaluation of the infant's respiratory status is paramount. There are no specific differences between ACP or PCP treatment.

En route to the hospital, the patient's dyspnea decreases and cyanosis is milder.

Treatment Continued

Oxygen should continue to be administered and respiratory assessment ongoing.

Differential Diagnosis

- Tetralogy of Fallot.

Test Your Knowledge

1. What are characteristic anatomical features of Tetralogy of Fallot?
2. What are the classic signs and symptoms of Tetralogy of Fallot?
3. What is the greatest threat to these patients?
4. What is the patient's ECG interpretation?
5. Without intervention, what might this hypercyanotic episode lead to?
6. Why do children with Tetralogy of Fallot squat or bring their knees to their chests?
7. Why do Tetralogy of Fallot patients rarely present with pulmonary edema?

CASE 25.2

Just after lunch on a warm summer's day, you are dispatched to 1022 Highway 10, Roland, Manitoba, for a possible childbirth. As you pull in the driveway and approach the house, you hurry to gather your equipment and obstetrics kit. You walk into the house and follow a woman's voice to the back bedroom, where she is on the bed and in the process of giving birth. You see that the baby's head has been delivered. You ask the woman to stop pushing while you assess the infant. She tells you she is 32 years old, that this is her first child, and that she is not due for another eight weeks. She has lost two other babies in miscarriages.

Initial Assessment Findings & Chief Complaint

LOA	Conscious and alert.
A	Patent.
B	Shallow rapid.
C	Strong radial pulses.
Wet Check	Bloody discharge from vagina.
CC	Childbirth.

History

S	Contractions leading to the delivery of the infant.
A	None.
M	None.
P	Three pregnancies, one infant, mother otherwise healthy, 32 weeks pregnant.
L	Breakfast.
E	The patient says she is 32 weeks pregnant and had a few irregular and infrequent contractions this morning. Right after lunch, the contractions became more regular and severe. She thinks her water broke this morning, but she is not sure as she was going to the bathroom. She wanted to drive to the hospital but the pain worsened. She called 911 and moments later started to give birth, just as you arrived.

Assessment

H/N	Unremarkable.
Chest	Unremarkable, with equal air entry bilaterally.
ABD	Contracting uterus.
Back	Unremarkable.
Pelvis	Stable.
Ext	Unremarkable.

Vitals

BP	128/68
P	80, irregular
RR	20
Pupils	PERL 3+ mm
GCS	4+5+6=15
BS	n/a
Pulse oximetry	98%
Skin	Cool, moist

Pain Assessment

O	n/a
P	n/a
Q	n/a
R	n/a
S	n/a
T	n/a

Cardiac Monitor

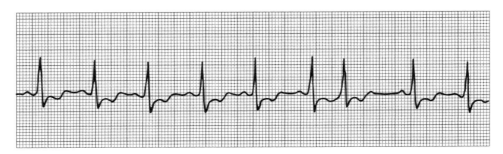

Figure 25.2

You assess the infant as the mother pants and is assessed by your partner. You observe the child's cyanosed head outside the vagina. You observe that the umbilical cord is not wrapped around the infant's neck. However, there is a thick, dark green substance in the infant's mouth.

Initial Treatment Post Assessment

The mother should be assessed and a complete set of vital signs obtained. Oxygen should be administered via a high concentration mask. An ECG interpretation should be completed. Your partner should stay with the mother and attempt to calm and facilitate communication between the two of you. An additional ambulance should be requested. After assessing the infant's mouth, you should attempt to suction the thick meconium from the infant prior to the continuation of delivery. Suctioning should be performed as you withdraw the catheter or bulb suction from the mouth or nose. Once the airway is clear, you should continue with the delivery of the infant on the next contraction. The infant should be wrapped and kept warm.

After the next contraction, the infant delivers and is cyanosed. The infant has shallow breathing and a heart rate of approximately 50.

Treatment Continued

The infant's airway should be reassessed for the presence of meconium, which should be suctioned if present. Ventilations and compression (120 per minute) at a breath-to-compression rate of 3:1 should be initiated on the infant for 15–20 seconds. After 20 seconds, the infant's pulse should be reassessed. If it is still less than 60, ventilations and compressions should be continued. If, after the first 20 seconds, there is no change in the infant's condition, an ACP should attempt to carry out an intubation and secure an ETT. Epinephrine 0.1 ml/kg should be administered via ETT using an appropriate technique, and can be readministered if warranted. The mother and infant should be transported to the nearest emergency department. Ongoing care for the mother and infant should be performed en route.

Differential Diagnosis

- Meconium aspiration.
- Neonatal resuscitation.

Test Your Knowledge

1. What is meconium?
2. What can meconium-stained amniotic fluid progress to?
3. Why is it important to remove meconium prior to stimulating the infant to breathe?
4. What suction level should be utilized when suctioning an infant?
5. Why is it important to keep the infant warm?
6. What is cold stress?
7. What occurs during cold stress?
8. What rhythm is the mother presenting with?

CASE 25.3

You are dispatched to 26 Rue Comeau, Caraquet, Quebec, for a possible one-month-old who is not breathing. As you pull up, the neighbour hurries you to the front door of the Leblanc residence. You are met by Clara, the child's mother, and handed the infant. It is 06:30hrs, and she tells you the baby, Yvon, went to sleep normally last night at 23:45hrs and that he usually wakes up at 06:00hrs. When he didn't wake up, she went to check in and found him not breathing. She tells you again that he was fine when he went to bed. The mother is sobbing and extremely upset.

Initial Assessment Findings & Chief Complaint

LOA	Unconscious, VSA.
A	Patent.
B	Apneic.
C	No brachial pulse present.
Wet Check	Unremarkable, diaper moist.
CC	VSA.

History

S	Unconscious, VSA.
A	None.
M	None.
P	Born at 38 weeks gestation without complications.
L	Breast-fed at 23:30hrs last night.
E	The infant was fed and put to bed in a bassinet beside the parents' bed. He normally fusses in the early hours, but did not wake up this morning. The father was working a night shift and left for work at 20:00hrs last night.

Assessment

H/N	Unremarkable, with mild cyanosis in lips and ears.
Chest	Unremarkable.
ABD	Unremarkable.
Back	Unremarkable.
Pelvis	Unremarkable.
Ext	Unremarkable, with mild cyanosis in hands.

Vitals

BP	0
P	0
RR	0
Pupils	5 non-reactive
GCS	1+1+1=3
BS	n/a
Pulse oximetry	0
Skin	Warm to touch, dry

Pain Assessment

O	n/a
P	n/a
Q	n/a
R	n/a
S	n/a
T	n/a

Cardiac Monitor

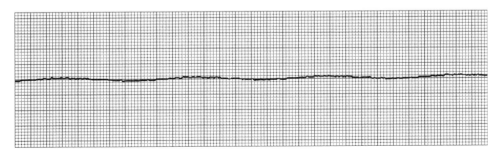

Figure 25.3

Initial Treatment Post Assessment

Initial treatment should include an assessment of breathing and circulation. CPR should be initiated and the infant transported to the waiting ambulance and to the hospital. The mother should accompany your partner in the front of the vehicle if dictated by local policy. An ACP should carry out intubation and verify and secure the ETT. Epinephrine and atropine should be administered via ETT every five minutes as per protocol. CPR should continue at the 3:1 ratio until arrival at the ER department. Because of transport times and a lack of personnel, an intravenous or IO may not be possible, and medication should continue to be administered via ETT.

En route, there is no change in the patient.

Cardiac Monitor

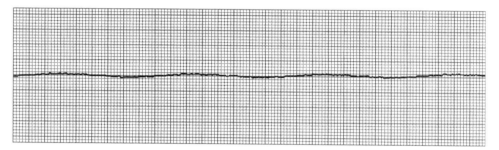

Figure 25.4

Treatment Continued

CPR should continue until arrival at the hospital, with a reassessment of the patient every five minutes.

Differential Diagnosis

- Sudden Infant Death Syndrome (SIDS).

Test Your Knowledge

1. What is SIDS?
2. At what age do most SIDS cases occur in Canada?
3. What is believed to cause SIDS?
4. Who is at risk for SIDS?
5. Who is at risk for an Apparent Life-Threatening Event (ALTE)?
6. What type of support should be available for the family of a SIDS patient?
7. Why might the infant still be warm to the touch?
8. What other process may be initiated by the death of an infant, only to compound the grief of the parents?
9. What is the interpretation of the patient's ECG?

Answers

Case 25.1

1. *What are characteristic anatomical features of Tetralogy of Fallot?*

    Tetralogy of Fallot is characterized by:

    Ventricular septal defect
    Dextroposition of the aorta
    Right ventricular hypertrophy
    Pulmonary stenosis

2. *What are the classic signs and symptoms of Tetralogy of Fallot?*

    The classic signs and symptoms of Tetralogy of Fallot include:

    Episodes of paroxysmal dyspnea with laboured respirations
    Cyanosis
    Possible syncope

3. *What is the greatest threat to these patients?*

    The greatest threat to these patients is a hypercyanotic episode, or "Tet spell."

4. *What is the patient's ECG interpretation?*

    The patient is presenting in an atrial tachycardia.

5. *Without intervention, what can this hypercyanotic episode lead to?*

    Without recognition and intervention, this may lead to complications such as seizures, lactic acidosis, cardiac arrhythmias, and death.

6. *Why do children with Tetralogy of Fallot squat or bring their knees to their chests?*

    The knees-to-chest position allows for increased venous return to the heart and an increase in systemic vascular resistance.

7. *Why do Tetralogy of Fallot patients rarely present with pulmonary edema?*

    CHF symptoms are rarely seen because blood is able to exit the right ventricle through the overriding aorta.

Case 25.2

1. *What is meconium?*

    Meconium is a dark green substance found in the digestive tract of newborns. It originates in various digestive glands.

2. *What can meconium-stained amniotic fluid progress to?*

    Inhalation of this thick secretion, either in utero or during an infant's first breath, can lead to aspiration and small-airway obstruction, which will lead to respiratory distress.

3. *Why is it important to remove meconium prior to stimulating the infant to breathe?*

    It is important to remove as much meconium as possible prior to stimulating the infant to breathe in order to prevent aspiration. Vigorous suctioning should occur before the baby has taken its first breath and while only the head is delivered.

4. *What suction level should be utilized when suctioning an infant?*

    The infant should be suctioned using a manual device such as a bulb suction. If a mechanical device is utilized, the vacuum level should be set to less than 100 mm Hg.

5. *Why is it important to keep the infant warm?*

   It is important to keep the infant warm in order to prevent cold shock. The infant has been incubated in a warm environment for many months, and entering a cooler environment will cause further problems post-delivery.

6. *What is cold stress?*

   Neonates are particularly prone to rapid heat loss because of their high surface-area-to-weight ratio. This ratio tends to be higher in neonates with low birth weights. Radiant heat loss occurs when bare skin is exposed to an environment with a cooler temperature. Since a neonate is wet with amniotic fluid, evaporation will lower body temperature.

7. *What occurs during cold stress?*

   Prolonged exposure without intervention diverts calories to produce heat. Neonates respond with sympathetic nerve discharge of norepinephrine in their brown fat. The reaction increases body temperature, but it also increases the baby's metabolic rate and oxygen consumption. With neonates in respiratory distress, cold stress may result in tissue hypoxia and neurological damage or metabolic acidosis and death.

8. *What rhythm is the mother presenting with?*

   The mother is presenting with an NSR with premature junctional beats.

Case 25.3

1. *What is SIDS?*

   SIDS stands for Sudden Infant Death Syndrome and is used to describe a syndrome of unexpected death in infants under one year, for which no pathological cause can be determined.

2. *At what age do most SIDS cases occur in Canada?*

   The peak incidence of SIDS in Canada occurs among patients two to four months of age.

3. *What is believed to cause SIDS?*

   There have been many theories of SIDS, but the most consistent appears to be infantile apnea, the exact nature of which is not clear. Dysrhythmias are usually the terminal event.

4. *Who is at risk for SIDS?*

   The following infants are at risk for SIDS:

   Term infants with an episode of an apparent life-threatening event
   Premature infants
   Low birth-weight infants
   Siblings of another infant who has died of SIDS
   Substance-abusing mothers

5. *Who is at risk for an Apparent Life Threatening Event (ALTE)?*

   Patients who demonstrate the following symptoms are at risk of an ALTE:

   Immature respiratory centre
   Chronic hypoxemia
   Sleep apnea with pallor or cyanosis
   Prolonged expiratory apnea
   Apnea related to an upper airway infection

6. *What type of support should be available for the family of a SIDS patient?*

   The family should be counselled and educated regarding SIDS. Since SIDS cannot be medically explained, the family is unequipped to prevent it in future. Parents may feel responsible and guilty for their infant's death. A hospital social worker or member of the clergy may aid in the support of the family at such time. Although an infant has died, the loss makes the family feel as if they, too, have been harmed.

7. *Why might the infant still be warm to touch?*

   The SIDS patient may be warm to touch because most infants wear full-length sleepers and are bundled in blankets to be kept warm at night.

8. *What other process may be initiated by the death of an infant, only to compound the grief of the parents?*

   Because SIDS infants usually die at home, they become coroners' cases. The police are generally involved in investigating the death to rule out foul play. This is an added stress to an already grieving family, who may feel guilty about the infant's death.

9. *What is the interpretation of the patient's ECG?*

   The patient is presenting in an asystole.

Chapter 26
Pediatrics

Tragedies involving children are often among the most stressful incidents of a paramedic's career. Pediatric treatment poses a significant number of challenges for paramedics, including communication barriers and inadequate patient history. Equipment challenges are also an issue, as most emergency medical equipment is designed for adults and modifications must be made for smaller patients. As well, the majority of incidents involving children are trauma-related. However, pediatric patients are transported infrequently, so exposure to children is minimal (unless you have your own). Practising good patient care and knowing treatment modalities for pediatric patients are important for paramedics. In the light of the high stress of pediatric calls, reliance on a solid foundation of pediatric knowledge is very beneficial. Remember, pediatric patients are not just small adults.

CASE 26.1

At 14:30hrs on a quiet summer day, you are imagining yourself relaxing by a pool on your next few days off. Your thoughts are interrupted by a call to 34 Shorncliff Avenue, Port Hardy, British Columbia, for an unconscious child. Your heart begins to race as you try to recall pediatric vitals and protocols. You have been a medic for many years and never look forward to "kid calls." As you arrive at the house, you are greeted by an elderly woman who tells you she cannot wake up her four-year-old grandson, Brodey. She further explains that he went to her room for a nap two hours earlier, and when she went to wake him she found him lying on the floor. She called 911 immediately. She appears scared and hesitant to answer questions as she tries to contact the child's father, who is at work.

Initial Assessment Findings & Chief Complaint

LOA	Unresponsive.
A	Appears patent.
B	Noisy respirations, snoring sounds.
C	Weak pulse at 60.
Wet Check	Unremarkable.
CC	Unconscious NYD.

History

S	Unconscious with shallow respirations.
A	None.
M	None.
P	None.
L	Breakfast.
E	After questioning, the grandmother tells you that when she entered the bedroom she found Brodey lying motionless on the floor. She also found her medication dosette beside him with pills on the floor. The labels on the dosette indicate that it contained metoprolol, glyburide, oxycodone, ECASA, and Vasotec.

Assessment

H/N	Trachea midline, no JVD, cyanosis in lips.
Chest	Unremarkable, but decreased air entry with transmitted upper airway sounds.
ABD	Soft/non-tender.
Back	Unremarkable.
Pelvis	Stable.
Ext	Normal, pale, with cyanosis in nail beds.

Vitals

BP	70/P
P	60
RR	6
Pupils	PERL 2- mm
GCS	1+1+1=3
BS	2.8 mmol/l
Pulse oximetry	86%
Skin	Pale, dry

Pain Assessment

O	n/a
P	n/a
Q	n/a
R	n/a
S	n/a
T	n/a

Cardiac Monitor

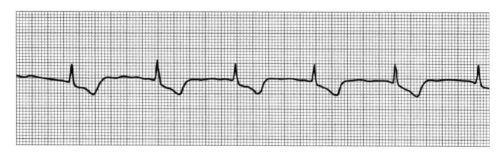

Figure 26.1

Initial Treatment Post Assessment

The initial treatment of Brodey should include assessment and control of his airway with an OPA and ventilations assisted with a BVM. A baseline set of vitals, including blood glucometry and an ECG interpretation, should be obtained. A complete assessment should be performed and the patient readied for transport to a hospital. An intravenous should also be initiated and a fluid bolus of 20 ml/kg started. Glucagon 0.5 mg SQ or approximately nine grams of D50W IV should be administered. If there is no change in the patient's level of consciousness, an ACP should secure the airway by intubation with an ETT no. 5, approximately 15 cm at the teeth, and confirm placement. Naloxone administration should be considered based on the patient's presentation and pupil size.

En route to the hospital, the patient has a generalized tonic-clonic seizure.

Treatment Continued

The child should be protected from the seizure, and as it continues, ventilation should be attempted to prevent hypoxia. An ACP should administer 4 mg diazepam. When the seizure subsides, the patient's airway should be reassessed and ventilation continued en route to the hospital. A repeat blood glucometry should be carried out because of the possible ingestion of glyburide. Assessment of the child should be ongoing. The IV bolus should be discontinued and run at TKVO if the patient's BP remains constant at approximately 100/P.

Differential Diagnosis

- Hypoglycemia.
- Narcotic overdose.

Test Your Knowledge

1. What is significant about the patient's position when you arrive on scene?
2. What ECG rhythm is Brodey presenting in?
3. What are the classifications of medications in the grandmother's dosette?
4. Based on your assessment, which medications has Brodey possibly ingested?
5. What are the typical milestones of development for a four year old?
6. What are normal vital signs for a four-year-old patient?
7. Is intubation of paramount importance in treating a pediatric patient?
8. What anatomical structures make intubation more challenging in a pediatric patient?

CASE 26.2

At 06:00hrs on a cold January morning, you are dispatched for a seven month old with difficulty breathing. You are approximately 10 minutes away from the address at 134 Macassa Circle, Kanata, Ontario. On arrival you are greeted by the mother, Lynn, who is holding her young son, Xavier. Lynn tells you her son has had a runny nose and congestion for the past few days. He started having trouble breathing around 05:00hrs and has since developed a loud, deep cough. You observe that the infant appears tired, is pale, and has mild cyanosis in the lips. As you enter the house, you hear the child coughing in a barking manner. The mother tells you that Xavier has been healthy since birth and is up-to-date on all his immunizations.

Initial Assessment Findings & Chief Complaint

LOA	Conscious, appears tired.
A	Patent.
B	Shallow, with audible stridor.
C	Strong brachial pulse present.
Wet Check	Unremarkable.
CC	Respiratory distress.

History

S	Patient is presenting with respiratory distress.
A	None.
M	Tempra drops.
P	Healthy child.
L	Last night, breast-fed prior to going to bed.
E	The mother states that the child has had what appeared to be a cold with a runny nose and fever over the past few days. Throughout the night, the child became restless and this morning had trouble breathing and started coughing.

Assessment

H/N	Cyanosis in the lips, with nasal flaring.
Chest	Accessory muscle usage inspiratory and expiratory stridor present.
ABD	Unremarkable.
Back	Unremarkable.
Pelvis	Stable.
Ext	Unremarkable.

Vitals

Pain Assessment

BP	Cuff too large for patient	O	n/a
P	150	P	n/a
RR	50 shallow	Q	n/a
Pupils	PERL 4+ mm	R	n/a
GCS	4+6+4=14	S	n/a
BS	n/a	T	n/a
Pulse oximetry	92%		
Skin	Pale, warm to touch		

Cardiac Monitor

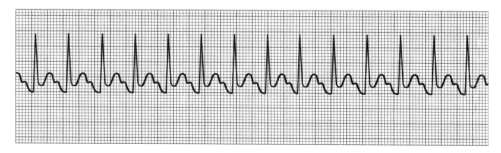

Figure 26.2

Initial Treatment Post Assessment

Initial assessment should concentrate on the respiratory efforts of the child. Oxygen saturation and a baseline set of vitals should be obtained from the patient, and an ECG interpretation done. Oxygen should be administered via a face mask or blow-by tube method with oxygen tubing. After an assessment, the patient should be wrapped in a blanket and carried to the waiting ambulance. Given the presence of respiratory distress and inspiratory and expiratory stridor, the patient should receive nebulized epinephrine per local protocol.

En route to the hospital, there is no significant change in the patient's condition and all vitals remain constant—with the exception of SPO2, which has risen to 94%.

Treatment Continued

A second dose of nebulized epinephrine should be considered, and supplemental oxygen administration should continue.

Differential Diagnosis

- Croup.

Test Your Knowledge

1. What is significant about the low, barking cough?
2. What is the classification of the medication being administered to the infant by the mother?
3. What is croup?
4. What are typical signs and symptoms of croup?
5. Is this condition generally a viral or bacterial infection?
6. What ECG is the patient presenting with?
7. What are normal vital signs for a seven-month-old infant?
8. What less invasive treatment can be utilized for a patient presenting with croup?

CASE 26.3

At 15:45hrs, you and another vehicle are dispatched to Highway 69 South, Sudbury, Ontario, just north of the Sergeant Rick McDonald Memorial Bridge for a vehicle pedestrian accident. Dispatch advises that the Ontario Provincial Police (OPP) are on scene and that there are two patients, both under 10 years old. On arrival you are met by a police officer, who reports that two brothers ran across the road after their dog and were struck by a small Mazda truck. Traffic has been stopped in both directions on the highway. As you approach the patients, you assess the first as VSA because his head appears to have been run over by the truck: grey matter and blood are scattered on the highway. The second patient is lying supine approximately three metres away, moaning and moving his left arm. He has obvious angulations of the right leg and arm and is in noted respiratory distress. He appears to be seven or eight years old. The second vehicle will care for the deceased on scene as you concentrate on the other young boy. The driver of the vehicle is not injured.

Initial Assessment Findings & Chief Complaint

LOA	Conscious but confused.
A	Patent.
B	Shallow, irregular respirations.
C	Weak femoral pulses are present.
Wet Check	Minor abrasions on chest, and laceration on right hip and forearm.
CC	Multiple trauma.

History

S	Altered level of consciousness, obvious trauma to the patient's right side.
A	CNO.
M	CNO.
P	MedicAlert necklace: asthma.
L	CNO.
E	Patient was crossing the road and was struck by a small truck at approximately 60 km/hr. His brother was also struck and is VSA on scene.

Assessment

H/N	No JVD, trachea is midline, abrasion on the right temporal lobe
Chest	Symmetrical with abrasions on entire right side of chest with equal air entry bilaterally.
ABD	Distended, with abrasions on right side of abdomen.
Back	Unremarkable.
Pelvis	Unstable.
Ext	Obvious simple fracture of right forearm and right femur, with poor capillary refill and absence of distal pulses.

Vitals

BP	72/66
P	45, weak, irregular
RR	36 shallow
Pupils	PERL 4 mm, slow to react
GCS	3+4+4=11
BS	n/a
Pulse oximetry	88%
Skin	Pale, cool, moist

Pain Assessment

O	n/a
P	n/a
Q	n/a
R	n/a
S	n/a
T	n/a

Cardiac Monitor

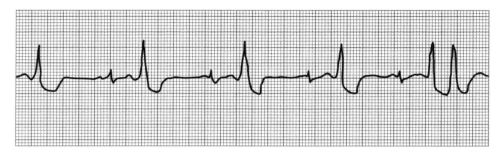

Figure 26.3

Initial Treatment Post Assessment

C-spine should be secured by your partner while a thorough primary assessment is completed. Since the patient is still responding and is maintaining his airway, adjuncts are not required at this time. Oxygen should be administered via a high concentration mask. A cervical collar should be applied and the patient secured to a scoop stretcher to avoid excessive movement of his unstable pelvis. Rapid transport to the hospital should be initiated, and minimal scene time taken. En route, an intravenous should be established and a fluid bolus initiated at 20 ml/kg. Re-evaluation of the patient's mental status and airway maintenance should be ongoing.

Differential Diagnosis

- Multi-system trauma.
- Hypoperfusion.

Test Your Knowledge

1. What is significant about the patient's injuries when you arrive on scene?
2. Approximately how much blood might the patient have lost, based on his presentation?
3. What is the best indication of perfusion in a child?
4. Why is a blood pressure reading not a significant finding in a pediatric patient?
5. What are signs of hypoperfusion in a child?
6. What specific organs are more commonly injured in pediatric patients than adults?
7. What is the patient's ECG interpretation?

CASE 26.4

You are dispatched to 42 Monsignor Melanson Road, Saint-Quentin, New Brunswick, for a child with trouble breathing. Because of your location when the call comes in, it will be approximately 15 minutes before you arrive. At the scene, you are frantically motioned into the driveway by a group of older women. You grab your equipment and enter the house with your partner. A woman calls for you to come to the bedroom quickly. As you enter, you see a young child sitting in a tripod position with shallow respirations and a steady stream of drool from his mouth. The mother, Karen, tells you that her six-year-old son Joshua came home from school looking very sick and complaining of a sore throat. She called 911 because he looked so bad and she was worried.

Initial Assessment Findings & Chief Complaint

LOA	Appears distant but conscious.
A	Patent with excessive drooling.
B	Shallow, tachypneic, occasional stridor.
C	Strong radial pulse.
Wet Check	Unremarkable.
CC	Sore throat progressing to respiratory distress.

History

S	Sore throat, difficulty swallowing, dyspnea.
A	Amoxil.
M	None.
P	Healthy.
L	Lunch at school.
E	Joshua came home from school with a sore throat, then became febrile with dysphagia and excessive drooling.

Assessment

H/N	No JVD, trachea midline, nasal flaring present.
Chest	Accessory muscle usage with shallow, equal respirations and occasional stridor.
ABD	Soft/non-tender.
Back	Unremarkable.
Pelvis	Stable.
Ext	Motionless, with decreased strength.

Vitals

BP	116/68
P	150
RR	40 shallow
Pupils	PERL 4+ mm
GCS	4+4+6=14
BS	4.8 mmol/l
Pulse oximetry	88%
Skin	Pale, hot to touch

Pain Assessment

O	n/a
P	n/a
Q	n/a
R	n/a
S	n/a
T	n/a

Cardiac Monitor

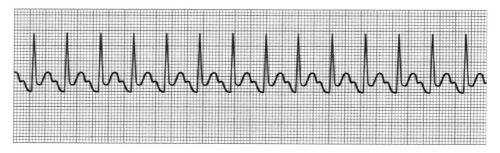

Figure 26.4

Initial Treatment Post Assessment

The patient should be assessed and vitals, including blood glucometry, should be obtained. Humidified oxygen should be administered via a face mask or blow-by tube technique. Ongoing cardiac monitoring should be maintained en route to the hospital. The patient should be kept calm and all attempts made to keep his anxiety to a minimum. The patient should be transported to the hospital without delay. There are no specific differences between ACP and PCP treatment. Should the patient become unconscious, then intubation may need to be carried out by an ACP. If possible, however, no attempts at intubation should be made in the field.

Differential Diagnosis

- Epiglottitis.

Test Your Knowledge

1. What is epiglottitis?
2. What are the typical signs and symptoms of epiglottitis?
3. What causes epiglottitis?

4. Who does epiglottitis affect?
5. What ECG is the patient presenting with?
6. Why should humidified oxygen be administered to a patient presenting with epiglottitis?
7. What should be avoided during an assessment of a child who may have epiglottitis?

CASE 26.5

You are dispatched on a warm fall afternoon to 36 Rue Fleurie, Pohenegamook, Quebec, for an eight-year-old child who has been burned by a pot of boiling water. On your way to the call, you think of your seven year old at home and imagine the agony the parents are going through. As you back into the driveway, you are greeted by the teenaged brother, who is crying. You think quietly, "This can't be good." He directs you to the kitchen where the child is being cared for by his mother. She is applying cold cloths to the boy's chest and back. She explains that there was a large pot of boiling water for canning on the stove. The boys were tossing a football in the house and the pot was accidentally knocked over, spilling on Michel, the eight year old. As you look for confirmation from the older brother, you see he is visibly upset and afraid. Michel is alert and presents with mild shortness of breath. He is only wearing shorts and visible blistering is developing on his back and neck.

Initial Assessment Findings & Chief Complaint

LOA	Conscious and alert.
A	Patent.
B	Shallow and fast.
C	Strong radial pulses.
Wet Check	Damp with water from the pot and towel application.
CC	Burns.

History

S	Complaining of pain from burns.
A	None.
M	Methylphenidate hydrochloride, dicyclomine, Serevent.
P	ADD, IBS, asthma.
L	Lunch.
E	Children were playing football in the house and accidentally knocked over a pot of boiling water on the patient. The cooling process was initiated immediately by applying cold cloths to the burns.

Assessment

H/N	No JVD, trachea midline, reddened area on anterior neck.
Chest	Equal air entry with mild expiratory wheezing, and redness over entire chest with blistering on upper chest across the nipple line.
ABD	Blistering over the entire abdomen with redness laterally.
Back	Blistering on both shoulders, and redness on the upper back bilaterally to the inferior scapulas.
Pelvis	Stable, but redness on groin, penis, and scrotum under the patient's shorts.
Ext	Redness on bilateral lower arms (anterior aspect) and on anterior aspect of right upper leg

Vitals

BP	106/72
P	120, strong and regular
RR	28
Pupils	PERL 3+ mm
GCS	4+5+6=15
BS	n/a
Pulse oximetry	97%
Skin	Warm to touch

Pain Assessment

O	n/a
P	n/a
Q	n/a
R	n/a
S	n/a
T	n/a

Cardiac Monitor

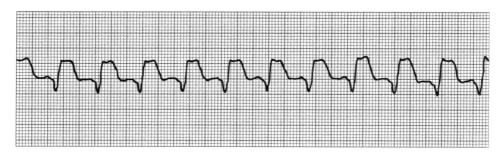

Figure 26.5

Initial Treatment Post Assessment

A primary assessment should be completed, including an assessment of the patient's respiratory status. All clothing should be removed. A baseline set of vitals should be obtained as well as an interpretation of the patient's ECG. Oxygen via a high concentration mask should be administered. As transport time will be less than 20 minutes, damp dressings can be applied to the burns. An intravenous should be initiated and run at TKVO. An ACP should administer narcotic analgesics such as morphine sulphate or fentanyl to help combat pain. Careful attention must be paid to the patient's vitals signs. Transport should be initiated promptly and the patient positioned as comfortably as possible on a stretcher.

En route, the patient has increased respiratory difficulty, audible stridor, and inspiratory and expiratory wheezing bilaterally. He is becoming more tired, and his BP has fallen to 90/60. His heart rate is at 100 bpm. You are approximately two minutes from the hospital.

Treatment Continued

Intravenous therapy should include initiating a 20 ml/kg bolus with evaluation of the lung fields for the presence of pulmonary edema every 250 ml. Nebulized salbutamol of 2.5–5.0 mg should be administered en route. Ongoing re-evaluation of the patient's airway is essential.

Differential Diagnosis

- Partial and full thickness burns, leading to hypovolemia and respiratory distress.

Test Your Knowledge

1. What is significant about the treatment Michel has received from his mother?
2. What is the total body surface area (BSA) of Michel's burns?
3. How does the BSA calculation differ between a child and an adult?
4. What classifications are the patient's medications?
5. What should paramedics be concerned about with Michel's upper chest and throat burns?
6. Should treatment of burns be based on transport time to a hospital?
7. What is the patient's ECG interpretation?
8. Based on your assessment, has Michel sustained minor, major, or critical burns? Why?

Answers
Case 26.1

1. *What is significant about the patient's position when you arrive on scene?*

    The patient is lying on the floor, which means he likely didn't go to bed two hours earlier but began playing with the medication dosette. This indicates that the medication may have been ingested some time ago.

2. *What ECG rhythm is Brodey presenting in?*

    Brodey is presenting in a junctional escape rhythm.

3. *What are the classifications of medications in the grandmother's dosette?*

metoprolol (Lopressor)	– Beta blocker
glyburide (Diabeta)	– Sulfonylureas, used to help control blood sugar levels
oxycodone (Oxycontin)	– Narcotic analgesic
ECASA (Aspirin)	– Platelet inhibitor
Vasotec (enalapril)	– ACE inhibitor

4. *Based on your assessment, which medications has Brodey possibly ingested?*

    Based on Brodey's unconscious state, shallow respirations, pinpoint pupils, and bradycardia, Brodey could have ingested Oxycodone, glyburide, and Metoprolol.

5. *What are the typical milestones of development for a four year old?*

The typical developmental milestones of a four-year-old (preschooler) include:

   Can run, walk, skip but has frequently associated injuries
   Imitates adult conversation
   May not be able to explain things, believing others see things from their viewpoint
   Thinking is literal and rooted in present time
   Thinks in absolutes (i.e., either good or bad)
   May not understand cause and effect
   Believes injury is punishment for bad behaviour
   Fears pain and separation from parents
   Older preschooler might make up symptoms

6. *What are normal vital signs for a four-year-old patient?*

   Normal vital signs for a four-year-old are
   BP: 98/65; systolic approximately 90 + 2x age; diastolic approximately 2/3 of systolic.
   P: 70–110 beats per minute
   RR: 22–34 breaths per minute

7. *Is intubation of paramount importance in treating a pediatric patient?*

   Airway management is extremely important, especially in pediatric patients. Recent studies have stressed that less invasive management is more appropriate. Insertion of an OPA and ventilation with a BVM, providing adequate ventilation and perfusion, is appropriate for pre-hospital care. Less emphasis should be placed on intubation in the pre-hospital setting, however, in order to reduce the complications of pediatric airway management.

8. *What anatomical structures of a pediatric patient make intubation more challenging?*

   The following characteristics of a child's anatomy may make intubation more challenging:

   Airway diameter is smaller and more easily obstructed
   Tongue is proportionally larger than jaw
   Epiglottis is floppier and more cephalid
   Larynx is more anterior and superior
   Infants are obligate nose breathers
   Airway structures are more flexible
   Mucous membranes are loosely attached
   Cricoid cartilage is narrowest part of funnel
   Trachea is shorter

Case 26.2

1. *What is significant about the low, barking cough?*

   The presentation of the low barking cough is a classic indicator of croup.

2. *What is the classification of the medication being administered to the infant by the mother?*

   Tempra (acetaminophen) – Analgesic, anti-pyretic

3. *What is croup?*

   Croup, or laryngotracheobronchitis, is an upper airway infection. Croup causes an inflammation of the subglottic area of the upper respiratory tract. The infection leads to edema beneath the larynx and glottis. The result is a narrowing of the airway lumen.

4. **What are typical signs and symptoms of croup?**

   The classic signs and symptoms of croup include:

   > The child usually presents with a cold or other infection
   > Usually occurs at night or early in the morning
   > Low grade fever
   > Hoarse voice
   > Barking cough
   > Inspiratory and expiratory stridor
   > Use of accessory muscles (chest in pediatrics)
   > Tachypnea
   > Tachycardia
   > Child prefers to sit up

5. **Is this condition generally a viral or bacterial infection?**

   Croup is a viral infection of the upper airway.

6. **What ECG is the patient presenting with?**

   The patient is presenting with a sinus tachycardia.

7. **What are normal vital signs for a seven-month-old infant?**

   Normal vital signs for a seven-month-old are:
   BP: Not usually measured in a child under three years of age, but systolic is 90 + 2x age
   P: 100–160 bpm
   RR: 30–60

8. **What less invasive treatment can be utilized for a patient presenting with croup?**

   During the trip from the residence to the ambulance, allow the patient to breathe cold outside air. The temperature of the air causes a reduction in the amount of edema in the subglottic region. During the short trip to the ambulance, the patient's breathing may improve dramatically.

Case 26.3

1. **What is significant about the patient's injuries when you arrive on scene?**

   The patient has sustained injuries to the entire right side of his body. He has sustained multiple traumas to the right chest, arm, and leg, as well as to his pelvis and possibly his head.

2. **Approximately how much blood might the patient have lost based on his presentation?**

   Based on the patient's presentation, he has lost 25–35 percent of his circulating volume.

3. **What is the best indication of systemic perfusion in a child?**

   The best indication of perfusion in a child is the presence and volume of peripheral pulses and the child's mental status.
   > Low-output shock: weak, thready, narrow PP
   > High-output shock: bounding, wide PP
   > Loss of central pulses is a premorbid sign; it heralds the approach of death.

4. **Why is blood pressure not a significant finding in a pediatric patient?**

   Blood pressure is not a significant finding in a pediatric patient because children will not tolerate respiratory failure or shock. Evidence of shock may be seen in tachycardia and poor skin perfusion or mental status. Children have excellent compensatory mechanisms, though it cannot be stressed enough that children's compensatory processes will eventually fail. As a young patient loses blood, his or her blood pressure plummets. Bradycardia, hypotension, or irregular respirations are extremely ominous signs of late shock.

5. *What are signs of early and late shock hypoperfusion in a child?*

Early shock:	Late shock:
Anxiety	Lethargy or coma
Tachycardia	Bradycardia
Tachypnea	Slow irregular breathing
Normal systolic BP	Hypotension
Weak peripheral pulses	Absent peripheral pulses
Delayed capillary refill	Markedly delayed or absent capillary refill
Pale extremities	Mottled extremities

6. *What specific organs are more commonly injured in pediatric patients than adults?*

   The spleen and liver are more commonly injured in children.

7. *What is the patient's ECG interpretation?*

   The patient is presenting in a sinus bradycardia with PVCs.

Case 26.4

1. *What is epiglottitis?*

   Epiglottitis is a life-threatening bacterial infection and subsequent inflammation of the epiglottis.

2. *What are the typical signs and symptoms of epiglottitis?*

   The typical signs and symptoms of epiglottitis include:

   Sore throat
   Pain on swallowing
   Shallow respirations
   Dyspnea
   High fever
   Frightened appearance
   Excessive drooling
   Pallor
   Inspiratory stridor
   Accessory muscle usage
   Sniffing position
   Nasal flaring
   Pulmonary hyperexpansion

3. *What causes epiglottitis?*

   Epiglottitis is caused by a bacterial infection; for example, Hemophilus influenza B.

4. *Who does epiglottitis effect?*

   Epiglottitis impacts children between the ages of three and seven, but is becoming less common as a result of the influenza vaccine in schools. The incidence of epiglottitis is increasing in the adult population.

5. *What ECG is the patient presenting with?*

   The patient is presenting with a sinus tachycardia.

6. *Why should humidified oxygen be administered to a patient presenting with epiglottitis?*

   The patient should be administered humidified oxygen to prevent drying of the epiglottitis and the airway.

7. *What should be avoided during an assessment of a child with the possibility of epiglottitis?*

    Assessment of the inside of the mouth or inserting anything in the patient's mouth should be avoided. Anything else that aggravates the child should be avoided, e.g., initiation of an intravenous.

Case 26.5

1. *What is significant about the treatment Michel has received from his mother?*

    The mother's quick thinking has provided a significant treatment to her son. By applying wet, cool cloths to Michel, she has stopped the burning process. This is important in the overall treatment of the patient.

2. *What is the total body surface area (BSA) of Michel's burns?*

Head/neck	Anterior neck	4%
Chest/ABD	Entire trunk	15%
Back	Upper back	8%
Arms	Anterior lower × 2	5%
Legs	Anterior upper × 1	5%
Genitals	Penis and scrotum	1%
Total:		38% BSA

3. *How does the BSA calculation differ between a child and an adult?*

    In an adult's BSA calculation, the Rule of Nines is utilized, assigning 9 percent to each of the 11 regions of the body and 1 percent to the genitals. In assessing BSA in children, this rule is modified to reflect the increased size of the head and the smaller size of the lower extremities. For an infant, it is further modified to reflect the infant's size.

4. *What classifications are the patient's medications?*

Methylphenidate hydrochloride (Ritalin)	– Mild central nervous system stimulant
dicyclomine (Bentylol)	– Anti-spasmodic
Serevent (salmeterol xinafoate)	– Long-acting inhaled bronchodilator

5. *Why should paramedics be concerned about Michel's upper chest and throat burns?*

    Paramedics should be concerned about the burns on Michel's upper chest and throat as they can lead to laryngeal edema and obstruction of the airway.

6. *Should treatment of burns be based on transport time to a hospital?*

    Wet dressings can replace dry dressings during short transport times.

7. *What is the patient's ECG interpretation?*

    Michel is presenting in an accelerated junctional rhythm.

8. *Based on your assessment, has Michel sustained minor, major, or critical burns? Why?*

    The patient's burns are considered critical as he has more than 20 percent BSA partial thickness burns and has also sustained full thickness burns. He also has burns to his perineum and face.

Chapter 27
Geriatrics

The gradual progression of age is a complicated process we will all experience. With the population aging and baby-boomers maturing, the vast majority of ambulance calls are becoming geriatric related. During the latter years of life, structural changes occur within the body that lead to systemic organ deterioration or failure. With this deterioration of systems, many signs and symptoms can be masked by other underlying problems. Compounding this, elderly patients tend to be on more medications than younger patients, and medications may also mask or have a synergistic effect on symptoms. As geriatric patients' hearing and sight diminish over time, patience and empathy should characterize all interactions with the geriatric patient.

CASE 27.1

It is a cold and blustery winter day when you are dispatched at 11:30hrs to 200 Foxforn Avenue, Elkhorn, Manitoba, for a collapsed elderly female. On arrival, you hear a cry for help from an elderly man inside the house. You enter slowly and he calls to you from the kitchen. As you approach, you see an elderly man kneeling on the floor with his wife's head in his lap. He introduces himself as Clarence and his wife as Ruth, and tells you that she collapsed while making lunch. He caught her and helped her to the ground. He tells you that he thought he had lost her, but that she is still breathing and opens her eyes on hearing a voice. She is weak and pale. Clarence says that over the past several months Ruth has been back and forth to the doctor getting new prescriptions to keep her blood pressure down. While preparing to cook lunch today, Ruth was having a glass of grapefruit juice, something she has every day, when she suddenly appeared to faint.

Initial Assessment Findings & Chief Complaint

LOA	Conscious, opens her eyes on hearing a voice, and whispers she is tired.
A	Patent.
B	Normal.
C	No radial pulses; carotid weak at 50 bpm.
Wet Check	Unremarkable.
CC	Syncope.

History

S	Weakness.
A	None.
M	NTG, digoxin, Adalat for the past month, Norvasc for three weeks, metoprolol for two weeks, HCT just started two days ago. All prescribed by the same doctor. The husband is not sure which medications the patient is or is not taking.
P	MI 10 years ago, angina, hip replacement, and ongoing attempts to use different medications to control BP.
L	Breakfast.
E	The patient was making lunch when she felt weak and dizzy and collapsed.

Assessment

H/N	No JVD, trachea midline.
Chest	Unremarkable, equal air entry bilaterally.
ABD	Soft/non-tender.
Back	Unremarkable.
Pelvis	Stable.
Ext	Weakness in all extremities, mild peripheral edema present in both ankles.

Vitals

BP	66/46
P	50, regular
RR	18 full volume
Pupils	Left & right somewhat reactive with cataracts
GCS	3+5+6=14
BS	4.8 mmol/l
Pulse oximetry	97%
Skin	Pale, diaphoretic

Pain Assessment

O	n/a
P	n/a
Q	n/a
R	n/a
S	n/a
T	n/a

Cardiac Monitor

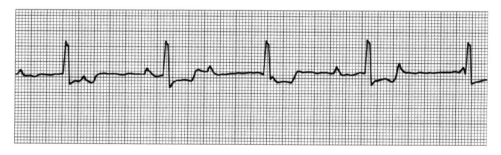

Figure 27.1

Initial Treatment Post Assessment

Initial treatment should include a thorough assessment of the patient. A complete set of vitals, including SPO2, blood glucometry, and an ECG interpretation, should be obtained. Oxygen should be administered via a high concentration mask. An intravenous should be secured and a 20 ml/kg bolus initiated. If there is no response with the fluid bolus, an ACP should initiate a dopamine infusion according to local protocol, and make preparations for external pacing. The patient should be transported in a non-elevated position on a stretcher and reassessed routinely en route to the hospital.

En route, the patient's blood pressure rises to 90/60 after 750 mls of IV fluid. There is no significant change in the patient's heart rate or rhythm. She tells you that she had a bout of chest discomfort and took three sprays of NTG prior to her collapse.

Cardiac Monitor

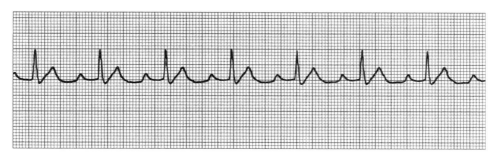

Figure 27.2

Treatment Continued

The intravenous bolus should continue, and an ACP should continue to administer dopamine and initiate pacing.

Differential Diagnosis

- Acute hypotensive crisis.
- Possible non-intentional overdose of cardiac-specific medications.
- Polypharmacy.

Test Your Knowledge

1. What is significant about the number of medications the patient has been prescribed to control her blood pressure?
2. What are the classifications of the patient's medications?
3. What ECG rhythm is the patient presenting in?
4. What is the patient at risk for while taking her current prescribed medications?
5. What else could be causing the reduction in blood pressure?
6. What may help the patient avoid a repeat of this situation?

CASE 27.2

At 15:30hrs, you are dispatched to the front of Blockbuster at the Kingsgate Shopping Centre in Vancouver for a female patient walking in and out of the parking lot traffic. As you pull up to the mall entrance, you observe an elderly female blocking the left lane. People in their cars are honking at the woman, who appears to be confused. You exit the vehicle and walk over to escort her out of the way of traffic. You introduce yourself and the woman walks with you. You observe that she is wearing her sweater inside out and that it is buttoned out of sequence. She appears otherwise well-dressed.

Initial Assessment Findings & Chief Complaint

LOA	Conscious, but appears confused.
A	Patent.
B	Normal, full volume.
C	Strong radial pulse.
Wet Check	Unremarkable.
CC	Confused.

History

S	The patient appears confused and lost in traffic.
A	CNO.
M	CNO.
P	MedicAlert necklace: Angina.
L	CNO.
E	The patient was observed walking in and out of traffic at a local mall parking lot. She appears to be alone and confused as to her surroundings. It is uncertain how long the patient has been on the premises.

Assessment

H/N	Unremarkable, no JVD, trachea midline.
Chest	Equal air entry bilaterally. An old midline surgical scar is present on the patient's chest.
ABD	Soft/non-tender.
Back	Unremarkable.
Pelvis	Stable.
Ext	Equal strength and mobility. No peripheral edema is present.

Vitals / Pain Assessment

BP	158/88	O	n/a
P	75	P	n/a
RR	16	Q	n/a
Pupils	PERL 3+ mm	R	n/a
GCS	4+4+6=14	S	n/a
BS	6.8 mmol/l	T	n/a
Pulse oximetry	97%		
Skin	Warm and dry		

Cardiac Monitor

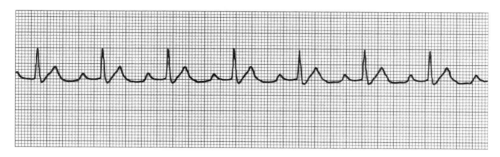

Figure 27.3

Initial Treatment Post Assessment

Initial treatment includes approaching the patient in a calm and non-threatening manner. She should be directed to the waiting ambulance for assessment. A complete set of vital signs should be obtained, including SPO2 and blood glucometry. Ongoing communication should be continued to discover where she is from and how she got there. Supportive care is important, as the patient appears to be confused about her surroundings. Once a conversation is underway, local police should be notified to aid with the patient.

Differential Diagnosis

- Possible dementia.

Test Your Knowledge

1. What is significant about the patient, her dress, and her level of awareness?
2. What is dementia?
3. List eight classifications of dementia, and include a possible cause for each classification.
4. What ECG is the patient presenting with?
5. If the patient has a history of dementia, what medications might you anticipate her to be taking?
6. What are the differences between dementia and delirium?

Answers

Case 27.1

1. ***What is significant about the number of medications the patient has been prescribed to control her blood pressure?***

    It is significant that the patient is on a high number of medications to control her blood pressure. In many situations, controlling a patient's blood pressure is purely a process of trial and error. Once the correct medication or combination of medications has been found, the patient remains on this prescription. However, a common error in carrying out this process is that patients are prescribed too many medications. The normal process requires that the patient discontinue previously prescribed medications before beginning the next trial. Elderly patients, however, may become confused and refill outdated prescriptions. The patient may thus remain on several medications in the same pharmaceutical category, putting him or her in a potentially critical situation. A sign that this has occurred in this instance is that the husband is not positive which medications the patient is currently taking, and that the patient has all the prescribed medication at home with her.

2. *What are the classifications of the patient's medications?*

NTG (nitroglycerine)	– Vascular smooth muscle relaxant
digoxin (Lanoxin)	– Cardiac glycoside
Adalat (nifedipine)	– Anti-anginal, antihypertensive
Norvasc (amlodipine)	– Anti-anginal, antihypertensive
metoprolol (Lopressor)	– Beta blocker
HCT (HCT)	– Diuretic

3. *What ECG rhythm is the patient presenting in?*

The patient is presenting in a third-degree AV block.

4. *What is the patient at risk for while she is taking the current prescribed medications?*

The patient is at risk of a severe hypotensive crisis. The combination of calcium channel blockers and beta blockers may pose a great risk of lowering cardiac output and pushing the patient to a more advanced stage of congestive heart failure.

5. *What else could be causing the reduction in blood pressure?*

Interestingly enough, the patient's daily routine involves drinking grapefruit juice, which interacts with calcium channel blockers. By inhibiting cytochrome 450, flavanoids present in grapefruit juice can increase plasma levels and augment effects of dihydropyridine calcium channel blockers. Grapefruit juice should therefore be avoided.

6. *What may help the patient avoid a repeat of this situation?*

The patient needs to have her prescriptions reviewed, and any medications not currently being taken should be discarded. The patient, with the aid of a pharmacist, can have her medications filled in a dosette that allows her to see daily what she is required to take.

Case 27.2

1. *What is significant about the patient, her dress, and her level of awareness?*

When the patient is initially observed in the parking lot, she appears to be confused and unaware of her surroundings and particularly of the potential danger to her personal safety. She is also wearing her sweater inside out and it is not buttoned properly, leading paramedics to believe she may have dressed herself and is under the care of someone or some residence.

2. *What is dementia?*

Dementia, a chronic global cognitive impairment, is often irreversible. It is often due to an underlying neurological disease called Organic Brain Syndrome.

3. *List eight classifications of dementia, and include a possible cause for each classification.*

Degenerative:	Alzheimer's or Huntington disease
Vascular:	Hypoperfusion
Infectious:	Meningitis
Inflammatory:	Systemic lupus
Toxic:	Alcohol- or medication-related
Metabolic:	Thyroid disease

Psychiatric:	Depression
Neoplastic:	Primary tumors

4. *What ECG is the patient presenting with?*

   The patient is presenting in a first-degree AV block.

5. *If the patient has a history of dementia, what medications might you anticipate her to be taking?*

   With dementia, it can be anticipated that the patient is taking some type of anti-psychotic medication.

6. *What are the differences between dementia and delirium?*

   Delirium tends to have a more rapid onset than dementia. It also impairs attention and focal cognitive function. Dementia, on the other hand, may alter memory, and the patient may present with global cognitive deficits. Furthermore, delirium requires immediate treatment and may be reversed, whereas dementia is usually a chronic condition.

Chapter 28
Abuse and Assault

Abuse and assault cross all socio-economic boundaries and transcend gender, race, and age. Although most assaults are associated with physical abuse, emotional abuse is also immeasurable and occurs just as frequently. Abuse and assault are most commonly viewed as occurring among pediatrics or couples, but in fact, the elderly are abused just as frequently as people of other ages. The most difficult aspect of abuse for paramedics is that its ill effects may often only be seen after many years. Paramedics should remember that they are the eyes and ears of the physician while on scene, and should pay particular attention to the physical surroundings of a home. They should also pay close attention to the demeanors of the patient and caregiver.

CASE 28.1

You are dispatched to 12 School Street, Montague, Prince Edward Island, for a possible fractured arm. On arrival, you are met by a father and his eight-year-old-son in the driveway. The young boy is supporting his right arm. The father tells you that the child, Adam, is clumsy and is always tripping. The father says he is very hyper and was running down the stairs when he tripped and fell. Adam is quiet and does not speak as the father discusses the accident with you. The father walks Adam toward the ambulance and tells you that he will follow you to the hospital. You open the side door and sit Adam in the jump seat to conduct your assessment.

Initial Assessment Findings & Chief Complaint

LOA	Conscious and alert.
A	Patent.
B	Regular and full volume.
C	Strong radial pulses.
Wet Check	Unremarkable.
CC	Possible fractured arm.

History

S	Pain and paresthesia in right lower arm.
A	None.
M	Ritalin.
P	ADD.
L	Breakfast this morning.
E	According to the father, Adam tripped and fell down the stairs. Once in the back of the ambulance, Adam is quiet and reserved. He is hesitant to talk about what happened. He finally tells you that he fell in the kitchen while getting peanut butter from the cupboard.

Assessment

H/N	Unremarkable.
Chest	Tender right lateral ribs with bluish and purple bruising. Equal air entry bilaterally.
ABD	Soft with slight tenderness in right flank area, with faint brown bruising.
Back	Large bruise (brown) on the right scapula, with mild pain on palpation.
Pelvis	Stable.
Ext	Equal strength and mobility in unaffected extremities, with some minor abrasions on the knuckles. The right wrist is angulated, with paresthesia present and good circulation and capillary refill.

294 Division 3 Other Emergencies

Vitals

BP	108/68
P	88, strong and regular
RR	20 full volume
Pupils	PERL 3+ mm
GCS	4+5+6=15
BS	n/a
Pulse oximetry	100%
Skin	Warm, dry

Pain Assessment

O	Sudden
P	Fall
Q	Constant ache
R	None
S	8/10
T	30 minutes

Cardiac Monitor

Not applied.

During your assessment, the patient is hesitant for you to look under his shirt. When asked about bruising, he tells you that he is clumsy and often falls.

Initial Treatment Post Assessment

Because of the patient's age, the initial assessment should be calm in order to make him comfortable. A thorough assessment should be completed and vital signs assessed. The possible fractured wrist should be assessed for the six Ps and splinted with a malleable or speed splint. The arm should be placed in a sling with a cold compress. An ACP may administer analgesics if within local protocol. Ongoing communication should continue en route to the hospital. Upon arrival, emergency staff should be made aware of your assessment findings and suspicions of child abuse.

Differential Diagnosis

- Fractured forearm.
- Child abuse.

Test Your Knowledge

1. What may be suspicious with regard to the demeanor of the child?
2. Based on the colour of Adam's bruises, how old might they be?
3. Why does this call raise suspicions of child abuse?
4. What is your obligation as a paramedic with reference to the possibility of child abuse?
5. What is the classification of the patient's medication?
6. As a paramedic, should you confront the father of the child?
7. In the patient incident history specifics, what might make you suspect abuse?

CASE 28.2

At 11:30hrs, you are dispatched to 1248 Bower Boulevard, Winnipeg, for an 85-year-old male who is weak and confused. As you arrive at the scene, you walk past suitcases to be greeted by a female approximately 60 years old. She directs you to the living room where Mr. Orlowski is sitting. He is wearing his pyjamas. She tells you that he is her father and needs to go to the hospital. She says he is weak and forgetful and needs to spend the weekend in a hospital to get better. She tells you that he has not been eating much and it is hard to leave him alone. The daughter appears anxious for you to leave with the patient. When asking for medical history and medications, she directs your partner to the patient's bedroom. Your partner observes a lock on the outside of the patient's bedroom door, a pail with approximately two litres of urine in it beside the bed, a bare, urine-stained mattress with one small blanket, and a garbage bag covering the window.

Initial Assessment Findings & Chief Complaint

LOA	Conscious, opens his eyes to your introduction.
A	Patent.
B	Shallow but regular.
C	Irregular radial pulse.
Wet Check	Dried urine on his pajamas.
CC	Weak, confused.

History

S	Increasing weakness and not eating.
A	None.
M	tacrine, sulindac, Restoril.
P	Glaucoma, mild dementia.
L	Yesterday evening.
E	The daughter states that her father has not been eating or drinking for several days and should go to the hospital. She said she cares for him but it is getting harder as he is uncooperative.

Assessment

H/N	No JVD, trachea midline.
Chest	Equal air entry, with mild wheezing present in the right lower lobe.
ABD	Soft/non-tender.
Back	Appears to have pressure sores on his lower back and buttocks.
Pelvis	Stable.
Ext	Unremarkable with weak grip strengths bilaterally, skin tenting, and poor capillary refill.

Vitals

BP	86/66
P	100, irregular
RR	20
Pupils	PERL 3+ mm
GCS	3+4+6=13
BS	4.8 mmol/l
Pulse oximetry	86%
Skin	Dry, tented

Pain Assessment

O	n/a
P	n/a
Q	n/a
R	n/a
S	n/a
T	n/a

Initial Treatment Post Assessment

The patient should have a complete assessment performed and a complete set of vitals should be obtained, including blood glucometry, SPO2, and an ECG interpretation. Oxygen should be administered via a high concentration mask at 12–15 lpm. An intravenous should be secured and a fluid bolus initiated. Salbutamol MDI should be administered if tolerated by the patient. The patient should be secured on a stretcher in a comfortable position and transported to the hospital.

Cardiac Monitor

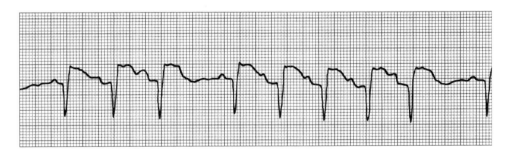

Figure 28.1

En route, the patient is resting and comfortable. His vital signs improve: BP 102/70, P 100, and RR 16. He still appears somewhat confused, but understands that you are taking him to the hospital.

Treatment Continued

The bolus should be discontinued and the IV infused at TKVO. Oxygen administration and supportive care should be continued during transport. Once at the hospital, concerns regarding the home life and living conditions of the patient should be addressed with the receiving physician, and followed up according to local policies.

Differential Diagnosis

- Dehydration.
- Possible elder abuse.

Test Your Knowledge

1. Based on your partner's assessment of the patient's room, why is there a distinct possibility of elder abuse in the care of this 85-year-old patient?
2. What appears peculiar with regards to the daughter's behaviour?
3. Is dementia the cause of the patient's decreased level of awareness?
4. What are typical signs and symptoms of neglect?
5. What classifications are the patient's medications?
6. What ECG is the patient presenting in?
7. What is a mnemonic useful in identifying elder abuse?

Answers

Case 28.1

1. *What may be suspicious with regards to the demeanor of the child?*
   The child appears quiet and reserved, allowing his dad to answer all questions. Although his father describes him as clumsy and very hyper, Adam is portraying the opposite. As well, Adam does not complain when his father decides to follow behind and not accompany him in the ambulance.
2. *Based on the colour of Adam's bruises, how old might they be?*
   Blue bruise on lateral ribs: 0–5 days old
   Brown bruise on flank/scapula: 10 or more days old
   Green bruises are often five to seven days old, yellow bruises are often seven to 10 days old, and usually, after two or more weeks, bruising clears.
3. *Why does this call raise suspicions of child abuse?*
   This call raises suspicions because of the physical bruising found in areas not typical of injury and the reluctance of the patient to allow you to assess his back and chest. It also raises suspicions that the father has a different story about how the son sustained the injury. The presence of a discrepancy in histories should prompt questioning.
4. *What is your obligation as a paramedic with reference to the possibility of child abuse?*
   If you suspect child abuse, you must report your suspicious findings to the receiving medical department. In some provinces, it is your legal obligation to report possible abuse to a child protective services agency or a government agency.
5. *What is the classification of the patient's medication?*
   Ritalin (methylphenidate) – Cerebral stimulant
6. *As a paramedic, should you confront the father of the child?*
   You should not make accusations or comments about your suspicions in front of the patient or bystanders. You should not try to cross-examine the parent but should obtain as much information as possible.
7. *In the patient incident history specifics, what might make you suspect abuse?*
   Evidence that may suggest abuse can be found in the validity of the history provided.
   Did the story change?
   Are the mechanisms of injury beyond the capabilities of the incident in question?
   Is there a history of recurrent injuries?
   Is there a lack of interaction between the parent and child?
   Does there appear to be a lack of concern toward the child's injuries?
   Is there inappropriate fear or lack of emotion?

Case 28.2

1. ***Based on your partner's assessment of the patient's room, why is there a distinct possibility of elder abuse in the care of this 85-year-old patient?***
   In the patient's room, many disturbing observations are made of things that would not typically be found in a person's bedroom. The first suspicious finding is the lock on the outside of the bedroom door. Since the lock is on the outside, it cannot keep the caregiver out; however, it can easily be used to lock the patient in the room. The second suspicious observation is the bucket of urine, which looks as if it is being used as a toilet. This is sometimes acceptable, as elderly patients may have difficulty getting to the bathroom, but a caregiver would normally provide a commode. At the very least, the urine should be emptied routinely; the two litres shows that it is not. The lack of linen and the appearance of the bed also indicate little care for the father in the room. As well, the window blacked out with a garbage bag suggests an intention to keep someone from seeing in or out, and keeps the room dark, which may be unpleasant for the patient. All of these observations raise the suspicion of mistreatment or elder abuse.

2. ***What appears peculiar with regards to the daughter's behaviour?***
   It is peculiar that the daughter seems rushed and adamant that her father spend the weekend at the hospital. She appears to lack concern for his health. The daughter's suitcase at the front door also indicates that she has plans to go somewhere.

3. ***Is dementia the cause of the patient's decreased level of awareness?***
   Dementia may cause the patient to have some level of altered consciousness, but the underlying causes are dehydration (hypovolemia) and hypoxia.

4. ***What are typical signs and symptoms of neglect?***
   The typical signs and symptoms of neglect may include:

   Bruises, hair removal, or restraint marks
   Habit disorders
   Antisocial without underlying cause
   Conduct behaviour
   Torn, stained, or bloody underwear
   Dehydration
   Poor hygiene/bedsores

5. ***What classifications are the patient's medications?***
   tacrine (Cognex) – Anticholinesterase
   sulindac (Clinoril) – NSAID
   Restoril (temazepam) – Benzodiazepine

6. ***What ECG is the patient presenting in?***
   The patient is presenting in a second-degree AV block, type 1.

7. ***What is a mnemonic useful in identifying elder abuse?***
   S   Screen
   C   Central injuries
   R   Repetitive injuries
   A   Abuse
   P   Possessive caregiver
   E   Explanation inconsistent
   D   Direct questions

Chapter 29
The Chronic Patient

Paramedics will be exposed to many patients, young and old, who live with a variety of impairments or disabilities. Many cope well with day-to-day life, while others experience hardship and require ongoing care. The key to treating patients with impairments or disabilities is to understand and recognize their special condition or needs in order to make accommodations for their proper care. The challenged or chronic patient may present with multiple ailments or a progression of disease. Many patients with terminal illnesses choose to pass away at home with loved ones instead of in a hospital room. Paramedics must respect their decisions and treat these patients in accordance with legal statutes specific to each province.

CASE 29.1

At 20:05hrs, you are dispatched to 165 Thatcher Drive, North Battleford, Saskatchewan, for a patient with difficulty breathing. On arrival, the driveway and street are lined with cars. As you enter the house, you are greeted by a man who tells you that his wife's mother, who is in the back bedroom, is having trouble breathing. He further reports that she is a palliative patient and is expected to pass away within a few days. She has a valid DNR signed by her oncologist and family doctor. You work your way around family members both in and outside the bedroom. The daughter approaches and tells you that her mother does not want to go to the hospital; her wish is to die at home. When you see the patient, she looks emaciated, frail, and jaundiced. She is on home oxygen via nasal cannula at 2 lpm. She appears winded, but makes eye contact with you as you enter the room. You introduce your partner and yourself, and she says hello.

Initial Assessment Findings & Chief Complaint

LOA	Conscious but slightly confused.
A	Patent.
B	Shallow at 22.
C	Strong radial pulses.
Wet Check	Unremarkable.
CC	Difficulty breathing.

History

S	Dyspnea throughout the day.
A	None.
M	Duragesic, MS Contin, Lasix, Slow-K, Pulmicort, salbutamol.
P	Liver cancer, asthma.
L	Ensure for supper.
E	The patient has been having increasing breathing difficulties since this morning. The family thought the patient was going to die, and because of her distress they called an ambulance.

Assessment

H/N	No JVD, trachea midline.
Chest	Symmetrical, equal air entry with bilateral inspiratory and expiratory wheezing, and consolidation of the right lower lobe.
ABD	Distended, with ascites.
Back	Unremarkable.
Pelvis	Stable.
Ext	Weak in extremities.

Vitals

BP	110/70
P	70, irregular
RR	22
Pupils	PERL 2+ mm
GCS	4+4+6=14
BS	6.1 mmol/l
Pulse oximetry	88%
Skin	Warm, dry

Pain Assessment

O	n/a
P	n/a
Q	n/a
R	n/a
S	n/a
T	n/a

Cardiac Monitor

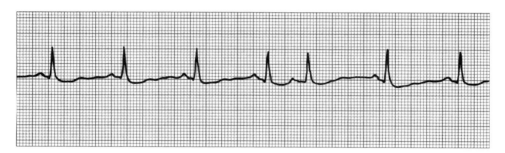

Figure 29.1

Initial Treatment Post Assessment

Empathy toward the family members should be demonstrated when you ask some of them to leave the room so you can examine the patient. Oxygen should be administered to the patient during your assessment. A complete set of vitals should be obtained, including SPO2 and blood glucometry. Palliative care patients will usually have nursing notes, which should be obtained and reviewed. Confirmation of the valid DNR should also be established, depending on local protocols for its acceptance. An ECG interpretation should be completed. Salbutamol should be administered via MDI or by nebulizer if MDI is not tolerated. The family should be advised of the patient's condition, and that she may benefit from being transported to the emergency department for further treatment. After further discussion, the patient should be placed in a position of optimal comfort. There is no significant difference in PCP or ACP treatment.

The patient agrees to go to the hospital, and her breathing improves with administration of salbutamol.

Differential Diagnosis

- Pneumonia in a palliative patient.

Test Your Knowledge

1. What legal versus ethical dilemma is faced by the paramedics on arrival at the residence?
2. What is your duty as you respond to the patient?
3. What is the paramedic's responsibility with regard to Do Not Resuscitate orders?
4. What are the classifications of the patient's medications?
5. Regarding terminal patients, what are the stages of death and grief?
6. What ECG is the patient presenting in?
7. What is meant by the phrase, "Do not resuscitate does not mean do not treat"?

CASE 29.2

It is just before quitting time when you are dispatched to 200 Clearwater Valley Road, Clearwater, British Columbia, for a patient choking and having difficulty breathing. On arrival you are greeted by Blaine, who tells you that his father, Daniel, appears to be choking and is having more difficulty breathing than he usually does. He tells you that Daniel has Lou Gehrig's disease and is in the bedroom, where he generally stays. As you enter the bedroom you observe the father, who appears to be approximately 60 years old, lying propped up by three pillows on a hospital bed. He is having moderate difficulty breathing and appears to be gagging. His son tells you that Daniel is unable to move from the neck down and can no longer speak. In order to communicate, he blinks his eyes in response to questions. You also notice a BPAP machine at the patient's bedside.

Initial Assessment Findings & Chief Complaint

LOA	Conscious.
A	Phlegm present in the patient's airway.
B	Laboured.
C	Strong radial pulses.
Wet Check	Unremarkable.
CC	Choking, dyspnea.

History

S	The patient has had an increase in phlegm and choking over the past few days and has been having more trouble sleeping.
A	None.
M	atenolol, Aldactone.
P	ALS, hypertension.
L	Lunch.
E	The patient had increased difficulty breathing throughout the day and more choking episodes.

Assessment

H/N	Unremarkable, no JVD, trachea midline.
Chest	Unremarkable, shallow respirations, with consolidation of the left lower lobe.
ABD	Soft/non-tender.
Back	Unremarkable.
Pelvis	Stable.
Ext	No mobility in extremities. Strong radial pulses present with normal capillary refill.

Vitals

BP	130/80
P	150, regular
RR	22 shallow
Pupils	PERL 3+ mm
GCS	Underlying 4+5+6=15
BS	4.8 mmol/l
Pulse oximetry	84%
Skin	Warm, dry

Pain Assessment

O	n/a
P	n/a
Q	n/a
R	n/a
S	n/a
T	n/a

Cardiac Monitor

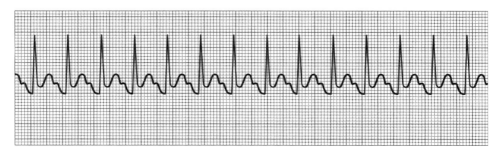

Figure 29.2

Initial Treatment Post Assessment

On arrival, the patient's airway should be assessed and suctioned. Oxygen should be applied via a high concentration mask post SPO2 assessment. A complete assessment should be performed. Vital signs, including blood glucometry and an ECG interpretation, should be obtained. The patient should be placed in a position to maximize air exchange. There should be communication with the son and father as to whether they have discussed advanced directives and whether a valid DNR order is in place. An intravenous should be established and the patient transported to the hospital. Continued care is the basis for ACP and PCP treatment.

En route, the patient appears more restless and dyspneic but maintains his oxygen saturations and level of awareness.

Treatment Continued

Routine evaluation of the patient's airway should be continually performed. Attempts at communication should be made throughout transport to ensure the patient's comfort. Communication will be challenging for both the patient and paramedic.

Differential Diagnosis

- Terminal effects of ALS.
- Pneumonia.

Test Your Knowledge

1. What is Lou Gehrig's disease or Amyotrophic lateral sclerosis (ALS)?
2. What are the typical causes of ALS?
3. What are the classifications of the patient's medications?
4. Despite profound motor impairment, what functions are usually spared?
5. What ECG is the patient presenting with?
6. Why does the patient utilize a BPAP machine at night?
7. What medications are used to prolong the lives of ALS patients?
8. What is the prognosis for Blaine's father, Daniel?

Answers

Case 29.1

1. *What legal versus ethical dilemma is faced by the paramedics on arrival at the residence?*
   Many of the patient's family members have gathered to show support for one another during a time of closure. They have accepted the fact that the patient wished to die at home. Now, however, paramedics have been summoned to help the patient in her increased distress. Many family members, as much as they have tried, have not prepared themselves for the increased distress the patient may have prior to passing. Effective communication and empathy toward family members will help them understand that while you respect their wishes, you must also assess and treat the patient. The patient has the legal right to a DNR order (in some provinces) and death with dignity. This is a choice made by the patient, usually in conversation with family members. However, most patients' passings are not as simple as movies portray, and the patient may experience increased distress prior to death. The apprehension of loved ones witnessing such distress sometimes causes family members to ask that paramedics intervene. Paramedics must follow provincial laws with respect to treatment regardless of the family's wishes or personal thoughts.

2. *What is your duty as you respond to the patient?*
   Your duty as a paramedic is to respect the patient's choices regardless of your morals or values.

3. *What is the paramedic's responsibility with regards to Do Not Resuscitate orders?*
   The paramedic's responsibility is to honour DNR orders when acceptable by law and local policy.

4. *What are the classifications of the patient's medications?*
   Duragesic (fentanyl) – Narcotic
   MS Contin (morphine) – Narcotic

Lasix (furosemide)	– Loop diuretic
Slow-K (potassium)	– Potassium supplement
Pulmicort (budesonide)	– Inhaled steroid
salbutamol (Ventolin)	– Bronchodilator

5. *Regarding terminal patients, what are the stages of death and grief?*
   The stages of death and grief include:
   Denial
   Anger
   Bargaining
   Depression
   Acceptance

6. *What ECG is the patient presenting in?*
   The patient is presenting in a normal sinus rhythm with premature atrial contractions.

7. *What is meant by the phrase, "Do not resuscitate does not mean do not treat"?*
   DNR patients may have complications unrelated to their terminal disease. These conditions should be treated regardless of DNR orders, as long as they do not require resuscitation.

Case 29.2

1. *What is Lou Gehrig's disease or Amyotrophic lateral sclerosis (ALS)?*
   ALS causes rapidly progressive muscle atrophy resulting from the degeneration of both upper and lower motor neurons. It causes varying degrees of spasticity, hyperreflexia, and muscle paralysis, leading to pulmonary complications. There is no cure for ALS.

2. *What are the typical causes of ALS?*
   The most likely cause of ALS is a genetic dysfunction of the enzyme superoxide dismutase causing responses to environmental insults. Cell death is a result of apoptosis.

3. *What are the classifications of the patient's medications?*
atenolol (Tenormin)	– Beta blocker
Aldactone (spironolactone)	– Potassium-sparing diuretic

4. *Despite profound motor impairment, what functions are usually spared?*
   Sensory and cognitive functions are usually spared.

5. *What ECG is the patient presenting with?*
   The patient is presenting with a sinus tachycardia.

6. *Why does the patient utilize a BPAP machine at night?*
   The patient uses a BPAP machine at night because of sleep apnea. Once accustomed to breathing through his nose and having his mouth closed, the patient's sleep apnea is diminished.

7. *What medications are used to prolong the lives of ALS patients?*
   riluzole (Rilutek) – Glutamate blocker

8. *What is the prognosis for Blaine's father, Daniel?*
   Daniel's prognosis is poor. In the end stage of treatment, patients may eventually consider forms of mechanical ventilation, such as a BPAP machine. This, of course, does not affect the progression of ALS.

Chapter 30
Nuclear, Biological, or Chemical Assault

Post 9/11, the world has become a different environment. This is nowhere more evident than in the day-to-day functions of emergency workers. Paramedics will be called upon for routine incidents, such as suspicious packages, as well as rarer events, such as possible chemical exposure. Emergency preparedness is the most important element available to paramedics in such situations. Self-protection and rapid intervention to limit exposure are key to the success of EMS intervention in a possible nuclear, biological, or chemical assault. As new smart bugs appear and the possibility of mass destruction grows, paramedics must stay current with treatment modalities, particularly in the prevention of contamination.

CASE 30.1

You are on standby during a peaceful student demonstration at the University of Saskatchewan when you are dispatched at 11:32hrs to a possible van explosion a block or so away. You proceed to the vehicle, reaching it in approximately four minutes, and find the minivan smouldering and the fire department on scene. Apparently, the explosion occurred 30 minutes prior. You see one male patient on the other side of the road talking to the fire captain. As you approach, you see that he has abrasions on his face, dried blood on his nostrils, and obvious burns on both hands. You escort him to the back of the ambulance. When asked what happened, he is hesitant, but tells you he was given $500 to drop the vehicle off at this address. When he started walking away, the vehicle exploded. He tells you that the van had canisters in the back, but he was unsure what was in them. You begin thinking of possible exposure hazards and don personal protective equipment. You observe that the patient is having respiratory difficulties. He tells you that his name is Wren and he is 20 years old.

Initial Assessment Findings & Chief Complaint

LOA	Conscious and alert.
A	Patent.
B	Shallow.
C	Strong radial pulses.
Wet Check	Unremarkable.
CC	Explosion.

History

S	Complaining of mild dyspnea with coughing, teary eyes, and pain in his hands.
A	None.
M	None.
P	Healthy.
L	Breakfast.
E	He parked the vehicle and was walking away when it exploded. He is complaining of mild difficulty breathing. He admits to doing nothing wrong and says he was just trying to make a few dollars. He now complains of nausea and his eyes are watering.

Assessment

H/N	Minor abrasions on face, dried blood on his nostrils, teary eyes.
Chest	Unremarkable, with equal air entry bilaterally and a non-productive cough.
ABD	Soft/non-tender.
Back	Unremarkable.
Pelvis	Stable.
Ext	Equal strength and mobility in all extremities, with first-degree burns on both hands.

Vitals

BP	126/86
P	72, irregular
RR	24 shallow
Pupils	PERL 3+ mm
GCS	4+5+6=15
BS	n/a
Pulse oximetry	94%
Skin	Warm and dry

Pain Assessment

O	n/a
P	n/a
Q	n/a
R	n/a
S	n/a
T	n/a

Cardiac Monitor

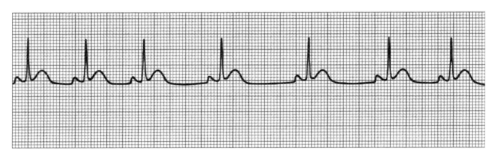

Figure 30.1

Initial Treatment Post Assessment

Initial treatment should include a complete assessment and vitals information, including SPO2 and ECG monitoring. Humidified oxygen should be administered via a high concentration mask and the patient should be placed in a position of comfort. The burns on his hands should be treated with wet saline dressings. An intravenous should be secured and infused TKVO. An ACP can administer narcotic analgesics intravenously for pain management.

En route to the hospital, the patient continues to cough and complains of painful eyes. His vitals remain stable.

Treatment Continued

Ongoing assessment of the patient should continue, as should irrigation of the burns. The patient's eyes can also be irrigated.

As you complete your call report at the hospital, the fire captain arrives and informs you that his team found canisters of chlorine in the back of the van.

Differential Diagnosis

- Burns on hands.
- Possible chemical exposure.

Test Your Knowledge

1. What precautions should be taken as you approach the scene?
2. What ECG is the patient presenting in?
3. What percentage of burns is the patient presenting with?
4. What type of agent is chlorine?
5. What are some possible signs and symptoms of chlorine exposure?
6. What may be the long-term signs and symptoms (occurring 12–24 hours later) of chlorine exposure?
7. What possible treatment might the patient receive?
8. What are the primary routes of exposure for chemical agents?

Answers

Case 30.1

1. *What precautions should be taken as you approach the scene?*

    As you approach, you should park upwind and take direction from the fire captain regarding possible contaminants or hazardous materials.

2. *What ECG is the patient presenting in?*

    The patient is presenting in a sinus dysrhythmia.

3. *What percentage of burns is the patient presenting with?*

    The patient has sustained approximately 5 percent burns on his BSA, particularly on his hands.

4. *What type of agent is chlorine?*

    Chlorine is a hazardous respiratory agent.

5. *What are some possible signs and symptoms of chlorine exposure?*

    Early signs and symptoms of chlorine exposure include immediate ocular and upper airway irritation as well as nausea and possible vomiting. Other signs and symptoms of more significant exposure include:

    Epistaxis
    Choking or coughing
    Stridor
    Tearing and painful eyes
    Nasal irritation
    Wheezing
    Substernal burning
    Dyspnea
    Suffocation
    Cyanosis
    Palpitations
    Syncope

6. ***What may be the long-term signs and symptoms (occurring 12–24 hours later) of chlorine exposure?***

   Within 12–24 hours, the patient may present with hoarseness, persistent coughing, and pulmonary edema.

7. ***What possible treatment might the patient receive?***

   Although controversial, the patient may receive nebulized sodium bicarbonate.

8. ***What are the primary routes of exposure for chemical agents?***

   The primary routes of exposure for chemical agents include inhalation, ingestion, and skin absorption or contact.